Bittersweet Baby

Jolie Kanat

CompCare Publishers
Minneapolis, Minnesota

Kanat, Jolie, 1952–
    Bittersweet baby.

    1. Kanat-Alexander, Sophie, 1984–   —Health.
2. Down's syndrome—Patients—United States—Biography.
3. Down's syndrome—Patients—Family relationships.
4. Kanat, Jolie, 1952–   —Diaries.   5. Mothers—
United States—Diaries.   I. Title.
RJ506.D68K36   1987   362.1'9892'858842   87-11657
ISBN 0-89638-123-4

Cover design by Kristen McDougall
Cover photo by Jaime Kanat

        Inquiries, orders, and catalog requests should be addressed to
        CompCare Publishers
        2415 Annapolis Lane
        Minneapolis, Minnesota 55441
        Call toll free 800/328-3330
        (Minnesota residents 559-4800)

This journal is
for every parent
of a child with a disability

Acknowledgments

Many people have been involved in my daughter's progress and have also seen me through some of the darkest months of my life. Here, at last, is an opportunity to thank them.

First and foremost I thank my irrepressibly optimistic husband, Peter Alexander, who has been Sophie's staunchest ally and my best, most beloved friend. My deepest thanks also:

To my mother, Doris Kanat, with whom I have mercilessly shared each loss and each milestone as they occurred. To my father, Walter Kanat, who is convinced that my daughter is the Princess of the World. To Sophie's brothers, Max, Moe, and Christopher, and sister, Becky—Sophie is lucky to have them. To Peter's parents, John and Charline Alexander, for their unconditional love and support. To my sister, Jaime Kanat, and brothers, Marc and Dean Kanat, for their sense of humor and excellent baby-sitting services.

To the doctors, counselors, and therapists who have treated and continued to care for my daughter—and me—with competence and concern: Jeffrey Birns, M.D., pediatric ear, nose, and throat specialist; Mary Coleman, M.D., pediatric neurologist; Ruth Lencione, Ph.D., director of the speech and language program for infants at California State University at Northridge; Andrew Matthew, M.D., pediatrician; and Bert Schoenkerman, M.D., my wonderful obstetrician and the first person to meet my beautiful daughter.

Also Robert Doman, Jr., president of the National Association for Child Development; Robin Millar, director of the Infant Stimulation program in Simi Valley, California; Bobbie Quigley, speech therapist extraordinaire; Kent Macleod, pharmacist and creator of the MSB formula, and Barry Pascal, pharmacist and developer of B_6 and magnesium in liquid form; Richard Bliss, D.C.; Ada Feldman, social worker; Sandra Meyer, director of correspondence education at the John Tracy Clinic in Los Angeles; Alfred Belleza and Tom Chandler, Scientology counselors; and Susan Gosnell and Robin Patton, physical therapy aids.

To Sophie's volunteers, Linda Bock, Bernie Brown, Renee Rosallini, Karen Whitely, and Laura Wittenberg, I thank you from the bottom of my heart for being there and for "just wanting to help."

To other parents, Brad and Glenda Boyajian, Ted and Suzanne Feit, Tim and Michelle Harrington, Bill and Adel Martin, and Jay and JoAnn Meepos and their incredible children, who have served not only as friends, but as partners, all of us learning as we go.

To Laura Gilbard and Bernie Brown and their magic word processors.

To my editor, Jane Thomas Noland, who managed to make my writing appear articulate and somewhat coherent, and to Margaret Marsh who made this book come true.

To Sophie, my little queen, who, against all medical predictions, will someday read this book.

And finally, to every person who said the right thing or who reached out to my daughter, ignoring the failings and applauding the successes. To every passerby, supermarket clerk, or elderly lady who exclaimed "What an adorable baby!" You made my day in ways you'll never know—and I'll never forget.

Contents

Foreword

Daily I am asked by a family with a child who has cerebral palsy, or brain injury, or Down Syndrome, or a learning disability, to recommend books which will help them understand their child. I usually cannot, because books have not been written about their child. Now I have one to recommend, for Jolie Kanat has written a book that is not about a disease, or a child who *is* a disease, but rather she has written a book about discovery.

Jolie and her daughter Sophie are fortunate, because Jolie as a parent was able to learn—in spite of professionals, institutions, and the ignorant—what most parents with children who are "special" may never have an opportunity to learn.

Somehow our enlightened, educated, God-fearing society has created a devastating myth surrounding a significant segment of our population. The myth is that some of us are not unique, that we are not miracles of creation, that we are instead "brain-injured," or "Down's," and, as such, without hope. The myth says that these children are not born with limitless potential and therefore should not be provided with open unlimited opportunities. These children are condemned from birth by myopic prejudice.

A "system," manned by an army of professionals is hard at work creating a "special" world for these children and future adults. "Special" programs for newborns and infants, "special" classrooms and schools, "special" training facilities and residences. These children are stripped at birth of their identities, their opportunities, and their futures.

Johnny Jones has brown hair and blue eyes. He loves animals and baseball. He hates school and broccoli. Johnny wants to be an astronaut when he growns up, and he has a little sister named Sue, whom he loves to torment. The myth turns Johnny into that child who *is* Down's, first, last, and foremost. He is simply one of those, defined only by Down's Syndrome. The "system" says, isn't it wonderful that we now know from birth how limited he is so that we can provide him with the appropriate "opportunities"?

Jolie discovered her daughter, her unique, loving, beautiful daughter, whose personality I suspect is very much like her mother's was at her age. Jolie's daughter, Sophie, is no longer a this or a that; Sophie is Sophie, unique, mysterious, and challenging, as are all children, and as with all children there is hope for the future. I suspect Sophie will never be "normal," not as defined by Webster as, "average, regular or standard"; Jolie would never stand for it. Sophie will, however, be given every reasonable opportunity to grow and develop as a member of her family and as a unique individual with limitless potential.

Jolie's journey of discovery was difficult, perhaps the most difficult of her life. But her discovery has rescued her daughter, and by rescuing her daughter she has saved herself. This arduous and often painful journey is one which needs to be made by every parent of a "special" child. For those of you who make this journey, your path will be easier, for now you have a guide who has been there.

Robert Doman, Jr.
President, National Association
for Child Development

Preface

In her autobiographical book, *Am I Getting Paid for This?*, Betty Rollin writes of an earlier book she wrote about her experience with cancer.

"If a person is going through some version of hell, it makes it easier, apparently, to hear or read about how someone else got through it—provided that person doesn't exaggerate, lie, or hide too much. People who are in a spot have a good nose for the straight story. They know when you're telling the truth and it can help them because (a) your truth is probably like theirs, so they feel less alone, and (b) they figure if someone as vain, uncourageous and ordinary as you got through it, so can they."

I think Ms. Rollin said it perfectly. When my baby was born, I needed to read a book for parents of children with disabilities—a book filled with honest emotions. I couldn't find one. I did find excellent books written in an inspirational, uplifting, positive, or educational manner. But I found none that shared the truth of pain and sorrow, of devastation and slow recovery on the part of the parents. How alone I felt!

Obviously not all of my personal experiences are shared by families with children like mine. However, I have tried to share enough of what we have gone through so that readers will recognize some common ground.

Our story is written in a journal format, as it happened and as I felt it. I was tempted to go back and "Monday morning quarterback it," filling in all my confusion and hurt with brilliant, insightful realizations. But I feel I would have cheated both myself and the reader.

If nothing else, I have learned through my recent experiences that just as you feel certain that you have a grasp of the "knowledge of life," a whole set of new truths may be thrown in your path.

This book is an account of my travels along that frustrating, confounding, sometimes rewarding, and—to me—remarkable path.

Introduction

My chubby ten-and-a-half-month-old daughter, Sophie, was playing in her crib this morning. Sweet, alluring baby sounds were coming from her room to ours as my husband and I lay half asleep.

It was my morning to wake up and make her a bottle. I stumbled groggily into her room. Even though I was sleepy and irritated at being awakened so early, my heart filled with joy at the sight of her. Her big blue eyes looked quickly up at me and her eager arms were raised high in the air to be lifted into a snuggly hug. I held her warm, kissable body close to mine, putting my cheek on her soft brown hair and one hand on a semi-soggy diaper.

Sophie's older brother was still sleeping, so I decided to take her quietly into our bed for her change and a bottle. I put her pint-sized body down on my big pillow and went to make her a bottle.

She looked so cozy and cute wedged between her sleepy papa and me as I fed her the warm bottle. At that moment I was feeling only satisfaction, affection, contentment, and a deep longing for more sleep. I felt none of the personal sorrow and pain that had assailed me in the past months. I was thinking how Sophie has put up with me through thick and thin, through my indecision, fear, anger, and endless sadness. She has seen me through confusion, helplessness, and apathy. She did not have the benefit of the confident, carefree Supermom that her big brother knew. Instead she tolerated me as an imperfect, tired, often frustrated mother, who was struggling to confront an impossible reality.

My daughter is no longer "a diagnosis." She and her brother are the light of our lives. Just seeing her beautiful face each morning is enough to brighten my whole day.

But this was not always so.

"Gold is a fine thing
For those who admire it.
Gold is like the sun
But I am a child
Of the moon, and silver
Is the metal of the moon.
Secret-smiler, wrapped in wonder,
Floating in her cloudy magic..."

lyrics by John Latouche
from the American opera,
The Ballad of Baby Doe

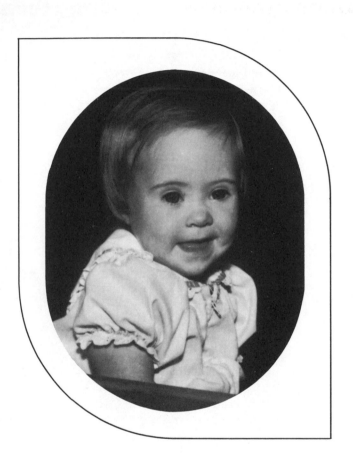

1

Down Syndrome—the words echoed in my mind like a scream down a tunnel

Thirty-one days ago, exactly one day short of nine of the longest months in the history of the universe, the labor pains for the birth of my second child began. It was 12:15 in the morning.

Since my first child, a boy, took approximately thirty-six hours to arrive, I felt confident that we had all the time in the world. Just one hour into the first labor pains, however, we were rushing to the hospital, hoping the baby would not be born in the back seat of my husband's brand-new family sedan. In the middle of one particularly excruciating contraction I remember thinking that he'd never forgive me if I wrecked his deluxe upholstery. Luckily we made it just in time. Our baby was born *au naturel* about forty-five minutes after we arrived at the hospital.

It was a painful but fast, relatively easy delivery. I wasn't even tired afterward. I was exhilarated and so proud of myself! I remember waiting anxiously for my obstetrician, Dr. Schoenkerman, to announce the sex of the baby. He seemed to be taking so long counting fingers and toes. He was uncurling the baby's hands and studying her palms. Finally the attending nurse cleared her throat and politely inquired, "Well, doctor, what do we have, a boy or a girl?"

"Oh!" My normally very alert and competent doctor seemed flustered. "Well! I forgot to look. It's a girl!"

A deep sigh of happiness and relief welled up inside of me. A daughter. A partner. My dream come true.

Even as Dr. Schoenkerman was examining her, my husband knew that, out of several names we had tentatively chosen, she was

a "Sophie." She was chubby, her coloring vivid—dark and rose.
Something about her shouted, "I am Sophie!"

As Dr. Schoenkerman handed her to me, he casually mentioned
that a line on her palm might indicate a "genetic problem." I
remember thinking, So he probably means her kids will inherit a
line on their palms—big deal, now give me my baby. Looking
back, I realize that the obstetrician showed remarkable restraint at
that moment. Later he told me that he "knew" immediately but
felt it was the pediatrician's place to make the diagnosis. By
waiting, he gave me the only time with my daughter that was
without stress and sadness for many months to come.

She was all wrapped up. She had lots of dark hair and her
cheeks were as red as beets. She was mine. She was spectacular.
She was perfect. At least for one more hour.

I immediately called my mother back East and left an excited,
happy message for her at work. Then I called my friend Raye and
bragged that I had a new daughter. (She was pregnant and really
hoping for a girl.) Right after those happy phone calls, I was
pleasantly surprised to see our pediatrician, Dr. Matthew, saunter
into our trendy Family Birthing Room, just about an hour and a
half after Sophie's birth. It's true he was a friend as well as our
wonderful and trusted pediatrician, but at 4:30 in the morning, this
was really above and beyond the call of duty! I didn't know then
that Dr. Schoenkerman had called him. Dr. Matthew was taking a
long time in the examining room with Sophie. My husband, Peter,
was tired and anxious to go home. My sister, who was taking care
of Sophie's three-and-a-half-year-old brother, Max, was waiting on
pins and needles for Peter to come home and tell her the good
news. At that point, neither my husband nor I had a clue that
anything was wrong. We just assumed Dr. Matthew was being his
usual careful self.

After about half an hour of waiting for him to finish the
examination, we decided it was best for Peter to go home, be with
Max, relieve my sister, and try to get some sleep. I didn't know
that, as my husband was walking down the hall, Dr. Matthew
waylaid him and asked him into the examining room. A little while
later, both my husband and Dr. Matthew returned to my room
looking really funereal—serious and very worried. I had never seen

my sweet, devilish husband looking so grave. The worried look included tentative glances at me to see if I was going to be able to handle what they were about to tell me. I was just hanging up the phone after bragging to someone else about my exciting new baby. I looked at them, thinking, Cheer up, guys—nothing's *that* bad; I saw the baby and she's fine, she's beautiful.

Both my husband and the doctor sat near my bed. Dr. Matthew began to state his observations—a line on her palm, a space between her toes (so far this did not seem like serious business), a fold of skin on her neck, extremely low muscle tone, upwardly slanted eyes, her slightly protruding tongue (it was starting to sound a little more disturbing now). He said that these symptoms were indicative of something called Trisomy 21.

The strange name did not ring a bell, so I was certain it must be something minor. The doctor was surely exaggerating the importance of these observations. Besides, I was sure this doctor—whom I had trusted completely up until ten minutes before—was imagining things. After all, it was very early in the morning and he hadn't had much sleep. I mean, nothing bad could ever happen to one of *my* children. But nonetheless I forced myself to ask, "By any chance, is there another name for this problem?"

"Yes," was all he offered.

"Well, what is it?" I asked bluntly.

I'll always remember the look of pain and hesitation on his face as he quietly answered, "Down Syndrome."

Down Syndrome—the words echoed in my mind like a scream down a tunnel.

At that very moment, the telephone in my room started to ring. I didn't want to answer it. I didn't know how to absorb this new information myself, much less share it with another person.

I lifted the phone, not knowing how I was going to sound. Was I going to be falsely cheerful? Hysterical? Secretive—not tell anyone?

It was my mother who, just an hour or so earlier, had received my happy message. "Hi, sweetie! So, is she gorgeous?" I could hear the excitement in her voice. "Yes, Mom," I kept my voice steady. "She looks just like Gam," I said, referring to my maternal grandmother.

Then, of course, my mother added immediately, "So, how did everything go? How are you? How is the baby?"

"Well, uh, Mom, there might be a problem." My voice seemed to be losing its steadiness.

There was immediate alarm in her voice, "What do you mean?" At that point, I wasn't totally prepared to accept the doctor's diagnosis myself; it was too new, too unreal. He had also told us that, although he was fairly certain, only a chromosome test could verify the evidence absolutely.

"Well, the baby might have Trisomy 21." I now knew why the doctor had used that medical term instead of the common one. It seemed so obscure, so safe.

"What's *that*?" I could hear the hesitation in my mother's voice.

"Mom, I, well, it's . . ." I couldn't say it. "Peter can tell you." I handed the phone to my tired husband and made him say what I could not. I felt cowardly but the words just would not come.

Peter told her straight, "The doctor thinks there's an indication that the baby has Down Syndrome."

The conversation lasted only about a minute more. After Peter hung up the phone, he told me she asked if we had just found out. He told her yes and she said she would give us some time and call back later. Peter told me she sounded pretty subdued. She told me some weeks later that, after the phone call, she had locked herself in the restroom at the school where she teaches and cried and cried.

I had the strangest feeling—the film reel was going in the wrong direction. We were supposed to be calling everyone we knew with the happiest news in the world. We were supposed to be looking forward eagerly to cheerful, present-laden visitors. I was supposed to be bragging about the easy delivery, the absolute beauty of my first baby girl. I was supposed to be nursing my baby, holding her chubby little body next to mine, filled with love, bursting with pride. Instead we were in a state of quiet shock and confusion. We had a million questions for the doctor. Would she live? How did this happen? What did this mean for the immediate future in terms of her health? Could we please hold her?

The doctor assured us that she had none of the heart problems commonly associated with babies with Down Syndrome and that we should watch for any potential intestinal problems like vomiting or lack of bowel movements. Because she was full term and weighed a healthy eight pounds seven ounces, he said she had a good start and, yes, we could hold her. He told us he would call a geneticist for a second opinion on her diagnosis but that he was fairly certain his observations were correct.

And so it began.

I didn't know what to do. I wasn't certain how to act. I'd never read a guidebook for a situation like this and neither had any of my family or friends. As much as I wanted to, I knew I couldn't keep this news a secret forever. Slowly I started making phone calls to friends and family members who had been anxiously awaiting news of the birth. After a few calls, I simply could not make that sad announcement one more time. I asked the nurse to bring me my baby, and I held her quietly for a while.

At 7:30 A.M. the geneticist came. He examined Sophie and shared his diagnosis with us. He told us unhesitatingly: Down Syndrome. Again he went over all the signs and symptoms, verifying what Dr. Matthew had told us. He said that although a chromosome test would verify the diagnosis it would simply confirm what he knew to be true.

✳ ✳ ✳ ✳ ✳

Never before can I remember being unable to stop crying. I cried the moment I woke up in the hospital the morning after Sophie's birth. I cried all through my unsuccessful attempts to eat breakfast. I cried through a phone call from my father. Here I was, thirty-two years old, and the last time I cried in front of my dad was when he punished me for putting my initials on my desk when I was seven. I think it really made my dad feel helpless, powerless to hear me so unhappy. I was irritated with myself for being so out of control.

Peter was at home with Max during much of this time. He had been pretty quiet about his feelings so far. We were both trying our best to hold it all together. We tried to be lighthearted when we were together in the hospital room, but we could hardly look at each other without being reminded of the pain inside us. We had failed. Out of our very happy and solid marriage came a little baby with problems so overwhelming we hardly knew what to think. But we both knew we had to function normally and carry on the best we could.

One of our first visitors at the hospital was my Aunt Dale. I tried to maintain a somewhat cheerful facade as I opened her baby gift—a frilly, pink, Polly-Flinders-style, aproned dress. It was tiny and perfect, just like my baby should be. But my baby wasn't perfect, and instead of cheering me up, the gift filled me with such a sense of loss and longing that I could barely look at it. At that point I knew I could not openly share how I felt with very many people. I mean, how would you feel if the person you'd just presented with a gift burst into tears at the sight of it? I was afraid that people would stay away, and I didn't want to start my daughter's life out that way. She already had enough problems.

During her first twenty-four hours of life, Sophie wasn't nursing well. Actually, she was sleeping through her feeding times, and I was worried. I called the nurse for some help. The nurse was like an Indian warrior! She unwrapped the baby and started pounding her feet, dancing her around the room and saying things like, "Sophie, wake up, it's time for lunch!" At first I was alarmed at all the rough handling, but I started to laugh when Sophie did wake up and show some interest in nursing. Soon I felt her tiny mouth tugging away at my breast. I felt like a mother again, not just a helpless bystander. If nothing else, I could at least offer my mysterious new baby this simple comfort and warmth.

✳ ✳ ✳ ✳ ✳

To attract pregnant couples, some hospitals these days offer such elegant amenities as our Family Birthing Room, which looked more like a deluxe hotel room. It had a canopied double bed covered with a peach chiffon bedspread. The room with its designer wallpaper was softly lit by color-coordinated matching lamps. There was a comfortable couch with colorful throw pillows for guests. Even the bathroom wallpaper matched the room's!

The hospital provided an elegant candlelight dinner for the new parents on the mother's last night there. I had waited nine long months for that special dinner and I didn't have enough sense to skip it this time around. Here is the usual scenario: The new young parents, flushed with pleasure at their mutual accomplishment, are guided down the hospital corridor to a private dining room. The room is lighted only by the flickering of two candles in sparkling crystal candlesticks. The candlesticks grace a beautifully set table, complete with pink tablecloth and fresh flowers. A bottle of iced champagne awaits the happy pair so they can begin their meal with a toast to their success.

It went a bit differently for us. My husband and I sat down. I had brought my foam doughnut pillow to sit on, for reasons known to all who have given birth. Peter raised his champagne-filled glass to mine and said, "To our family." I immediately burst into tears and continued crying from the shrimp cocktail through the cheese-cake. It was a soggy meal. I was so completely heartbroken.

Immediately after that endless meal we had an appointment in my hospital room with the geneticist who would answer our questions. To tell the truth, I was in no mood to see anyone, especially someone who was about to tell us his predictions for our baby's future. I wanted to crawl into a corner and die rather than put on a pleasant front, posing, along with my husband, as coherent adults facing a subject that, at this point, we weren't sure we wanted to learn about at all.

But the doctor was very considerate to come at that late hour, so Peter and I put our feelings aside. We asked him first about Sophie's physical health. He reassured us that, as ironic as it sounded, we had "a perfectly healthy baby with Down Syndrome." For that we were relieved and grateful.

Peter then asked about our daughter's future intellectual develop-ment. Respecting the doctor's credentials—he was not only a pediatrician but also held a Ph.D. in genetics—we hung on his every word.

He began to pace as he expounded, "Your daughter may never learn to read or write. Her IQ will probably reach thirty-five or so, at best. However there are manual labor workshops where perhaps she can be taught the simple tasks required to assemble manufac-tured parts." This last part was meant to cheer us up in case we were thinking she wouldn't be able to make a contribution. Mind you, our daughter was less than twenty-four hours old. It was bizarre and shocking, to say the least, to picture our tiny newborn in these future circumstances.

The doctor had more to say, but I was in such total shock at what he had just told us that I have no memory of the rest of the conversation. I only know that, two minutes after he left, visiting hours began and my room immediately filled with friends and family anxious to see the baby and to offer confused congratulations.

I'll tell you, I've had better days.

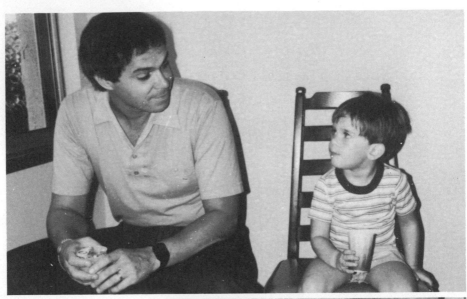

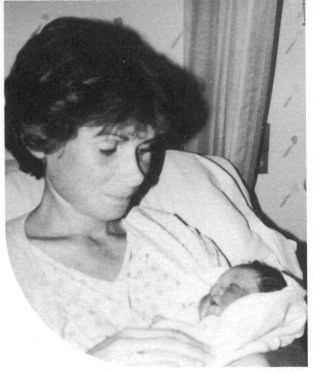

2

Secretly I wanted to lock the doors and pull down the shades

October 13. Sophie is four weeks old. I'm wondering if a day will ever go by when I don't cry, when I don't feel someone has reached into my carefree, happy life and pulled a shade down halfway.

One thought swirls endlessly in my head: how could this have happened to us? Or to Sophie? We are so normal, so perfectly suburban. We did everything right: we were a little older than most when we married; as time went by my husband got better and better jobs; we bought a tract home in a safe neighborhood to house our growing family. I was so careful with my pregnancies—not one sip of alcohol or caffeine. Not even an aspirin or a cough drop for fear it would somehow harm the fetus. During my pregnancy with Sophie, I didn't even lift my grocery bags; to avoid any strain on the baby, I paid neighborhood kids a quarter each to carry them from the car. As things turned out, I probably could have had a wild cough-drop orgy or tangoed with several heavy grocery bags all at once. It wouldn't have mattered.

I crossed over from one state of being into another after Sophie's birth. When I see pictures of myself pregnant with her, they seem to have been taken long ago, in another, simpler time. I feel so changed. I have become less intense, and many things seem less important to me. It's as if a fine shellac has melted off me and I'm rough around the edges. I just don't care so much about perfection anymore. Mine or anyone else's.

As much as I have tried to avoid it, I know that Sophie's big brother, Max, needs an explanation about his sister's problem. He's been hearing us talk about it and I'm sure he is curious and confused. I want him to have as much comprehension as possible

of the situation without narrowing or defining his future relationship with his sister in a negative way.

So today I assigned myself that sad task. I sat with Max in his
room on his "big boy" race-car bed, and I tried to explain why all
the extra fuss was being made over Sophie.

"She was born with a problem and we need to help her out a
little. It's called Down Syndrome. Can you say that, sweetie?"

My heart cracked in two when I heard his little three-and-a-half-
year-old voice say, "Down Syndrome."

"Good," I said, reassuring him that he had said it correctly.
Then I added, "And that's why sometimes I'm sad."

"You're sad because Sophie has a problem?" he asked in a very
serious voice.

"Yes, sweetie. But I'm okay and Sophie is fine. She just needs a
little of our time and help. And there are ways you can help too.
We'll teach you." I paused, looking at his face to see that he
seemed calm and interested. "Do you have any questions?" I
asked, wanting to make sure he was handling this new information
well.

"No," he answered casually, probably anxious to get back to his
toys.

"Okay." I gave him a kiss and left his room. I knew there
would be lots of future opportunities for other questions.

October 16. When Max was born there were not enough pots to
put the flowers in during my short hospital stay. They just kept
coming—plants, bouquets, balloons. I felt that the whole world
wanted to say, "Congratulations!"

With Sophie, there was a time lag on the arrival of the flowers, as
if people were momentarily stunned at the news and didn't quite
know what to do. When we came home from the hospital the
flowers started to arrive en masse. It felt strange, kind of halfway
between a birth and a funeral. Lots of gifts arrived too, even from
family and friends who had already given us presents at a baby

shower. Almost too many gifts. Consolation prizes. And visitors kept coming. Secretly I wanted to lock the doors and pull down the shades, but I knew I couldn't. I wanted to tell people, "Can't you see I am in mourning? Can't you see I am overwhelmed by grief? Just go away!" How could they understand that fully? I could hardly understand it myself.

3

I wish I weren't so uncertain about things that are so important

October 17. About two and a half weeks ago, I began to learn about the network of parents and educators involved with children with Down Syndrome. While in the hospital I had contacted a physical therapist from the Infant Stimulation program in my city. She answered many of my questions, suggested I get Sophie started as soon as possible, and asked if she could give my name to other parents of young children with Down Syndrome in the area. I'd forgotten about that part of the conversation until I received a call from a mother of a two-year-old daughter with Down Syndrome. During our talk, she mentioned a doctor in Washington, D.C., who was conducting a research program with infants who had Down Syndrome. The infants had to be less than six weeks old to participate. She gave me the doctor's number and address. I figured it was worth a call, although I had no idea how we'd get to Washington on such short notice if, indeed, the doctor were interested in our daughter and we were interested in the doctor's program.

The doctor, a world-renowned developmental specialist in autism and Down Syndrome, told us she would have to see the baby before *three weeks* of age, that there was no guarantee the program would be successful for our daughter, and that the necessary tests and examination could only take place in Washington. It didn't sound too promising, but we hadn't heard of any other, better alternatives to help our child. It took us about fifteen minutes to decide. We would go to Washington as soon as we could figure out how to pay for the flight. The moment we mentioned the project to our respective parents, they offered to help with plane fare and medical expenses.

We got Max situated at Peter's parents' house for the few days we'd be gone, packed a few things, made hotel, car, and flight reservations, bundled up the baby, along with hundreds of disposable diapers, and we were off! Not until we were in our seats on the plane and Sophie was asleep in my husband's arms did it hit me that this was not a fun family vacation. We were not just whisking off on the spur of the moment to the south of France for a little fun in the sun. But I was proud of myself. I only cried through half— not all—of the flight.

In the past when I had envisioned visiting our nation's capital, I had imagined a whirlwind sightseeing tour, covering all the hot spots—the monuments, the museums, the fine restaurants. Children's Hospital had not been on my list, but there I was, watching my daughter's tiny head being wired for something called a Brain Stem Evoked Potential test that had been ordered by Dr. H.*, the research physician whom we had come to see.

We sat with Sophie in the darkened soundproof audiologist's room. All wired up, she was sleeping in a sterile, steel hospital crib, while the technician flashed lights and sounds at her. How I wanted to grab her and run away from that place! She was too tiny and new to be put through such sophisticated and high-tech scientific testing. She looked like a baby robot.

Earlier, we had waited in one of the hospital lobbies until the lab technician was ready to give Sophie the blood test Dr. H. had ordered. After we had been sitting there a few minutes, a mother and her teenage daughter with Down Syndrome walked in and sat down next to us. Seeing the young girl was a shock for me. She was about sixteen years old, of average height, but she walked with an irregular gait. Her eyes were slanted and a bit crossed. Her legs seemed to be a little misshapen, and her speech was throaty and difficult to understand. She was well behaved but childlike in attitude.

Although I had to become aware of some of the realities of my daughter's condition at some point, I would have chosen a different

---

*The research physician, who requested anonymity to protect the privacy of her research at this time, is referred to throughout the book as Dr. H. (not her real initial).

moment. As a new mother, I'd had very little sleep in the past two weeks, and I was under stress the likes of which I had not known could exist. After a few minutes, Peter decided to walk around the halls with Sophie. I'm glad I wasn't holding her right then, because I started to cry uncontrollably and she would have needed a raincoat to protect her from my tears. I didn't even have a Kleenex in my purse. How could I have known that I would be crying in public at the drop of a hat? So I sat there, afraid to move, embarrassed to be seen. I was stuck in my seat with a runny nose and puffy eyes.

Finally we were called in for Sophie's blood test. Although she cried a little bit, all in all she was a real trooper—holding up much better than her mother.

We were relieved to escape the confines of the hospital and drive through the magnificent fall colors of several elegant Washington neighborhoods on our way to Dr. H.'s office—even though I was so preoccupied that I hardly enjoyed the passing scenery. I was anxious to meet the doctor, to discover what kind of a person she was and exactly what was in store for our baby.

Dr. H.'s office was located in a charming old house near a long block of foreign embassies. We were greeted by her assistant and asked to wait in a large room devoid of such frills as paintings or furniture, other than the couch we sat on. While waiting, we both lapsed into our private thoughts, which were interrupted by the doctor's entrance. She looked so—well, *smart*. I can't describe her any other way.

Once we were in her office, Dr. H. gave Sophie a most detailed exam, asking us at least one hundred questions and answering at least that many for us. She was very knowledgeable and reassured us that many of our fears were unfounded. She told us not to concern ourselves too intensely with Sophie's physical development, that it might be a little delayed but would come in time. She explained that her main concern was improving intellectual develop-ment. She had dedicated the past twenty years of her life to this.

Why, I wondered, would this woman choose this field of endeavor? She had worked for *years* in order to help children that most other professionals in the field had decided were simply always going to be the way they were. We were unspeakably grateful. We knew that we had found a lifelong ally.

During years of research and study, Dr. H. had discovered when newborn babies with Down Syndrome were given the Evoked Potential test, which measures the brain's ability to receive visual and audio stimuli, the results were always normal, provided there was no congenital blindness or deafness. If the babies were tested again after three weeks of age, the test results would always worsen. The current research program in which Sophie was about to become a participant was Dr. H.'s attempt to normalize the test results permanently by administering certain vitamins or thyroid medications to balance the child's metabolism. According to Dr. H., autopsies have shown no brain abnormalities or damage in people with Down Syndrome. Based on this evidence, she theorizes that the problems result from metabolic imbalances. What effect normalizing the Evoked Potential will eventually have on the child's intellectual and social development remains to be seen as the brand-new research project continues over time.

This is a thumbnail sketch of a complex subject, but to us it made enough sense to give it a try. The thing that really clinched it for us was that Dr. H. raved about how pretty our baby was. Now *that* we understood!

We left her office feeling buoyant—like parents again instead of victims of something we couldn't change or improve. A day or two after we returned home, we learned from Dr. H. that Sophie's blood test results showed that she had a normal thyroid level, normal Vitamin A and carotene. What she exhibited, however, was low serotonin, a neurotransmitter found in the bloodstream that induces constriction of the blood vessels and muscle contraction. Dr. H. explained that serotonin is the only brain chemical of its type that can be measured in the bloodstream. To raise the level of serotonin in Sophie's system we were to give her liquid Vitamin B_6 and magnesium every day in steadily increasing doses, which Dr. H. would prescribe for us as Sophie's weight increased.

We found a wonderful pharmacist who agreed to make the B_6 and magnesium in the exact form required by Dr. H. It is normally not available in liquid form. The taste of B_6 falls somewhere between old lemons and rotten eggs and getting Sophie to swallow it is a trick. Since she refuses the bottle and insists only upon nursing, we have to give her the mixture straight in a dropper. Getting it all down her is a struggle and sometimes I have to try two or three times before she actually swallows it. I can't wait until she is old enough for solid food.

So much has happened in four days! I took Sophie to her first day of Infant Stimulation, located in the rehabilitation section of a local hospital in a brightly painted, toy-filled room. Carrying my tiny new baby into that room was one of the bravest things I've ever done. I didn't cry. I was even coherent. I kept thinking that I was supposed to be at home instead, gossiping with friends and showing off our babies. This strange environment was all so new and unwelcome.

Sophie's first evaluation was private and lasted an hour and a half. The physical therapist tested every testable aspect of a month-old baby's development, and then some. She suggested I bring Sophie in once a week, to start, and we would begin to work on whichever areas needed attention.

As I drove home, instead of feeling glad that such a progressive program existed in my own city, I was depressed. I had not envisioned starting my baby's life in this way. And how was I going to balance out Max's needs and his schedule with his sister's?

I'm still feeling depressed, and I'm concerned about how Max is going to handle having his kingdom disrupted, not just by an intruder but by one with so many extra needs.

Today Sophie screamed as an audiologist gave her a second tympanogram. Dr. H. had recommended she get her ear fluid tested because she is always so congested. The doctor explained that, because of the Down Syndrome, Sophie's ear canals would not drain fluid well, leading to ear infections and possible hearing loss.

The tympanogram came out flat. The audiologist told me this means either that there's fluid in her ear or that she's too young for the results to be accurate. Great. Because her first tympanogram a week and a half ago also came out flat, she just finished ten gruesome days of a pink antibiotic that made her throw up every other time she took it. That, on top of her attempts to spit out the horrible-tasting B$_6$, is an upsetting way to start the day.

Already Sophie has three pediatricians, a developmental specialist, a physical therapist, and an audiologist, and she's just over a month old! I feel as if I'm torturing her. Should I just forget all of this running around and treat her like a regular kid? And who knows if any of these treatments will do any good? It seems so unnatural to be scheduling a tiny tot with all these therapists and tests and doctors. Is it all doing more harm than good? Maybe, instead, I'll just stay home and watch "The Price Is Right," with a half-gallon of fudge ice cream to keep me company.

Yesterday the president of the Down Syndrome Parents' Group told me that the chance of people with Down Syndrome getting leukemia is ten times that of the normal population. I guess things could always be worse.

I learned something else today. Apparently many children with Down Syndrome have severe speech delays and difficulties. This was a new piece of information. The therapists in Sophie's Infant Stimulation program use sign language for commonly used words like "eat" or "more" or "cracker" in order to help the kids communicate their needs if they're having trouble talking at an appropriate age. This way, explained the therapist, they don't become frustrated at their inability to let someone know what they want.

When I first saw the therapists signing to the kids, I was angry. Wait a minute! She's got enough problems, I thought, but she's not deaf! And, even if she *were* deaf, isn't sign language considered a lesser priority than teaching oral skills? And doesn't signing discourage speech? But after it was explained to me that the signs are used only until the children can replace them with words, I relaxed a little.

So now, of course, I'm wondering if I should take a sign language class so that I can start to sign immediately to Sophie. By doing so, would I be admitting or predicting that Sophie won't talk at an appropriate age? I'm not willing to accept that possibility right now. Or is it smart to afford her every opportunity to communicate as early and as effectively as possible? Sometimes it's difficult to decide what would be best for Sophie, regardless of whether or not *I* like the idea. The question of whether or not to learn sign language is just one example. Another is the physical therapy program. If I get depressed taking her to physical therapy (Infant Stimulation), should I ignore my feelings and tell myself that it is not for me, it is for her? Or should I go with my intuition? I wish I weren't so uncertain about things that are so important.

4

Who appointed me grand marshall
of this whole parade?

October 18. This afternoon I read an article in a well-known
magazine about a woman who, through an ultrasound exam,
discovered she was going to have twins. Through amniocentesis it
was also discovered that one of the twins had Down Syndrome.
Her medical "success story" was that her doctor was able to abort
the fetus with Down Syndrome and keep the other twin alive.

I was filled with a shivery horror at the thought of this. How my
own mind and heart have changed! A few months ago I might
have thought this was clever medicine. Now I can't help but feel
that this is a comment on the value of my daughter's life and on the
value of life itself. I believe much of the medical community feels
that a child with Down Syndrome is not worth granting life to, that
it would have been acceptable to have terminated the life of my
daughter rather than allow her to be born. And who knows how I
would have felt had I known beforehand. I have to confess that
although I feel strongly that abortion is ending life, I may have been
swayed by popular opinion regarding affirmative results of an
amniocentesis and opted to abort. I can only say that I am
eternally grateful that I have never had to face that decision. Can
you imagine giving birth to a child you loved with all your heart in
the midst of opinion that the child should have been aborted?

Since all my friends have healthy kids, I have no one to talk to
about issues like these. For the past three and a half years I've
surrounded myself with moms of kids my son's age. I've lived the
standard lifestyle of a first-time mother: attending Mommy and Me
classes, trying to find baby sitters, learning what to feed my son
other than peanut butter. These were life's big challenges. Max is

brilliant, beautiful, bratty, and big. He is crabby and energetic, a serious negotiator—in short, every mother's first "perfect" child— and I fully intended to go on having one or two more just like him.

Now I'm lost.

Sophie's potential problems have become bigger that she is. I'm more familiar with her chromosomal patterns that I am with her personality. She is just four and a half weeks old, and I've hardly had a moment to just be her mom.

✳ ✳ ✳ ✳ ✳

I've heard that the City of Hope Medical Center is starting a long-term research program on Down Syndrome. Apparently this is quite a step forward on a somewhat neglected subject. They're looking for infants to examine and follow over a long period of time to study treatment and therapies, and to observe for the first time the developmental patterns of a large number of children with Down Syndrome.

The president of the Down Syndrome Parents' Group says I should take Sophie to the City of Hope, if only to support the project. One of Sophie's pediatricians says I should go there because the doctors in the program are reported to be the best in each of their fields.

So, dutifully, I have made an appointment at the City of Hope. The program's administrator told me on the phone that there would be a two-day evaluation with several specialists examining my daughter. Appointments are during the day, so Peter will be unable to accompany me. I'm dying *not* to go. I know it will be awful and medical and probing. I know it will put a temporary strain on my sanity and on Sophie's well-being.

Again I'm uncertain. Should I brush all this aside and take her anyway because a team of physicians will then pay close attention to my daughter's development, and besides, lending my daughter to "science" for a couple of days to help future children is the right thing to do? Or should I just refuse to subject my baby to this scrutiny? This is all so new to me! It's like a hurricane in my life with no time to adjust to the fact that it's here and it's blowing my house down.

Then there are the friends and relatives. They mean well, but they don't seem to know quite what to say. Well, neither do I. After all, who appointed me grand marshall of this whole parade?

October 19. Peter has two children, Chris and Becky, from a previous marriage. They are thirteen and eleven. Today they met Sophie for the first time. I was concerned that they would be intimidated in some way by knowing that their half-sister was born with a problem. I had written their mother a note telling her, and I knew that she would have discussed the situation with the kids.

Well, the kids were great. Becky immediately fell in love with Sophie and wanted to change her diaper and hold her and see if her doll's clothes fit her. Typical of most thirteen-year-old boys, Chris pretty much ignored her except to say she was adorable. Then he quickly returned to his most recent Dungeon and Dragon strategies.

I realized that kids rarely have the preconceived notions that adults have and rarely do they harbor the same fears and judg-ments. I suppose they'll have time to learn them later on. But by then Sophie will just be Sophie to them and they'll treat her as they would any other mischievous little sister.

October 20. Another visit to Sophie's physical therapy class. There were two other mothers there with their babies. One five-month-old had Central Core Disease, a form of muscular dystrophy. He had purple surgical scars all over his small body from a recent opera-tion, and his color was pale blue because of a congenital heart defect. He was lying on one of the blue and yellow gym mats that covered the floor. The therapist was helping him with exercises to facilitate use of some of his muscles. The other mom had an eighteen-month-old daughter, who was really pretty but very still. The therapist explained to me that because this otherwise healthy child had seizures every seven seconds, her medication was causing her to be fairly inert. She had to be fed with a syringe, did not speak or seem to respond in any visible way. Seizures every *seven seconds*! Why *that* little girl? Why *that* mother? It's so devastating to be a witness to these uninvited complications in the lives of babies.

I can't handle this. Sometimes I feel my life is ruined, my future darkened. I can't seem to pull together. I now know the official definition of "falling apart." Sometimes I feel as if my mind is an overloaded circuit and I forget how to have a regular conversation. I've forgotten how I used to be.

While in line at the supermarket today with a monster load of groceries, holding Sophie in one arm and listening to my son as he launched into a major tantrum with all the trimmings, I started to shake him and shout at him to stop. The checker gave me a reproachful look that said, "What an abusive mother!" I felt like one, too. I wanted to say to her, "Look, lady, I can't explain right now but I'm going crazy and I'm sorry that you're seeing this. Just give me a few months and maybe I'll be okay. But right now you and I are not living in the same world."

I feel like an eggshell. I could be crushed at any time by the least pressure. My baby daughter was born with Down Syndrome and I'm frightened and sad and all predictability seems to have flown from my days.

✳ ✳ ✳ ✳ ✳

If I hear one more time how "happy these children are," I might just punch out the person who says it. Happy is nice, but what about sharp, witty, sexy, married, talented, clever, rich, and the mother of three? What about shopping for clothes for her high school valedictorian speech? What about planning her wedding together? I know these thoughts are pointless and selfish, but I have them nonetheless. They haunt me, chase me.

Will I eventually learn to accept Sophie and be content with exactly who she is? All I can think about right now is what she will never be. So what kind of a mother am I? I don't want to take my daughter to therapy or to doctors or to research programs. The situation is a nightmare. I don't want to be a "special mother." I want to be regular, and I want my baby to be regular. Is it wrong to think I'll die if I don't have a healthy daughter upon whom I can bestow every fantasized expectation? Is it wrong to be unable to adjust to something that is impossible to accept?

Suggestions on what to say to parents who have just given birth to a child with a disability

When Sophie was born and we were still in the hospital, so many friends and relatives told me they felt helpless and uncertain about what to say. Should they be happy about the new baby? Or sad? Or both? For them and for you I offer these guidelines for the future, should you ever encounter the situation. You can't go wrong with:

1. "What a beautiful baby!"

2. "How was your labor and delivery?"

3. "She's got your coloring."

4. "Congratulations!"

5. "Where can I set these flowers?"

I'm not saying that you should pretend that the problem doesn't exist. What I'm suggesting is that, first and foremost, there's a brand-new baby here and that fact needs to be acknowledged in a loving, considerate way. Remember that the mother just went through nine months of pregnancy, during which time she had at least one baby shower, bought furniture for a perfect nursery for her child's happy entrance into the world, abstained from chocolate, coffee, and liquor, went through several hours of hard labor, and was just told her baby had an irreversible genetic or physical disorder. The best thing you can do at that moment is to offer these parents simple normalcy and kindness.

Feel free to show sincere concern or to ask gentle questions about the baby's health. If the parents want to cry, don't tell them that everything's going to be okay. If they don't want to cry, don't feel insulted that they're not sharing their feelings with you. They may be feeling okay at that moment. Or perhaps the feelings are too raw to share.

On the other hand, just in case you have the following comments on the tip of your tongue during your hospital visit, keep them to yourself forever:

1. "Didn't you have amniocentesis?" Think about this question for a moment.

2. "God chooses special parents for special babies." As well-meaning as that statement is, at this sensitive point in the parents' lives it might tempt them to kick you *and* God out of their lives for quite a while.

3. "These children are always so sweet." All of a sudden, this brand-new baby has lost her individuality and has become grouped with a bunch of kids the parents have never even met. It is a child's personality—not a child's disability—that makes him or her sweet. A disability makes a child disabled. Some disabled kids are sweet, and some are hell on wheels—just like all kids.

4. "What exactly *is* Down Syndrome?" (or spina bifida or cerebral palsy, or whatever the problem may be). Remember, these people are new parents, not doctors. Chances are they're just learning the facts themselves. Repeatedly discussing their baby's medical prognosis can get depressing. Instead do a little research or ask someone else a few questions before going to visit. That way, your basic questions will be answered, and you'll be a lot more comfortable with the subject. Perhaps later on the parents will be able to discuss the subject more easily.

The parents know that you mean well. And most likely whatever you say will be met with kindness and gratitude, just because you're there and showing support. The best approach, if you can, is to place yourself for a moment in their shoes. What would *you* like someone to say to *you*?

5

Our hopes are high

November 1. Last weekend Peter and I attended a fascinating seminar on various rather unorthodox treatments for children with Down Syndrome.

Presenting their ideas were a panel of highly experienced specialists, including two doctors, a nutritionist, a chiropractor, a representative for a treatment called cell therapy, and the head of the National Association for Child Development (NACD). By the time we left we had learned so much that our heads were spinning with new thoughts and decisions to make.

Dr. Henry Turkel, a physician, presented amazing data on a treatment he had developed specifically for people with Down Syndrome. It consists of medication called the U-series. Dr. Turkel's theory is that children with Down Syndrome, because of their metabolic complications, do not process waste properly. He contends that deposits build up in the cells and organs of the body causing mental and physical delay and disfiguration. He showed before and after photographs of kids who had been on the U-series and they all looked markedly improved after treatment. He stated that the improvements, both mental and physical, were due to the U-series, which had helped to flush out trapped wastes in the body. He was very convincing, even though the Federal Drug Administration (FDA) had repeatedly refused to approve his treatment as valid.

Although we needed to research his claims further, we both felt that we wanted to look into the cost involved and talk to parents who had children being treated with U-series. We were amazed that, if his claims were true, they were not better known and more widely accepted.

A pediatrician spoke about the chronic congestion of many kids with Down Syndrome. Our ears perked up because congestion has been a nonstop problem with Sophie, causing ear infections, ear fluid, and possible (although we're not certain) partial hearing loss. This doctor suggested a nutritional approach, along with standard treatment with antibiotics.

A well-known nutritionist told how megavitamins had helped.

A chiropractor talked about the odontoid process, adjusting a section of the spine near the neck, to improve the physical development of children with Down Syndrome in order to avoid a somewhat common complication called atlanto-axial subluxation.

A parent of an autistic child presented a film on cell therapy. This treatment utilizes the injection of fetal cells of lambs to facilitate cell maturation in people who, for one reason or another, do not have proper cell growth. According to the information presented, in the case of children with Down Syndrome it is the brain cells that do not grow properly, although, according to Dr. H., the brain structure itself is not damaged by the chromosomal anomaly of Down Syndrome. The film focused on a Dr. Franz Schmid, who runs a clinic in Germany. He, too, reports great success during his twenty-five years of using this therapy. He claims the cells increase brain growth and improve functions of many other organs in the body. According to Dr. Schmid, the therapy has almost no side effects. Just one little catch. Cell therapy is not legal in the United States. You must either fly to Germany or find a doctor willing to risk his or her license (if you can somehow get the cells from Germany) to give your child the injections.

Of all the theories we have heard so far, this seems the most unusual. As intriguing as this program was, we were not ready to run out and buy our plane tickets to Deutschland. We still have some thinking and questioning to do.

The man who impressed us the most was Bob Doman from the National Association for Child Development. He offers a home program designed to improve both intellectual and physical growth for all children, not just for those with disabilities. The NACD publishes reports containing the organization's research and recommendations. One report, *The NACD Concept*, explains the group's fundamental premise: "The development of a child is neither random nor accidental . . . the genetic makeup of the child does not determine the level of function the child will ultimately obtain.''

In another report, *The Down's Syndrome Child*, Bob Doman writes: "The range of function found in Down's children is extremely broad. You cannot really make any generalized statements that are applicable to these children, as they would only serve to stifle and hinder their developmental growth. Historically and traditionally, Down's children have been placed into Trainable Mentally Retarded (TMR) classes and provided with the very minimum of what could be a truly developing educational atmosphere. Most research indicates that Down's children who stay in the home and who have been exposed to normal environmental stimuli function at a much higher level than those placed in special education environments. Without question, one of the most significant aspects of instruction for these children is to keep them in *normal environments*. This often means *excluding* them from the so-called special education programs, and the social organizations for special children which actually only serve to further isolate and stigmatize them. We attempt to either place them in a normal school situation, *or to keep them out of the formal school environment* [emphasis is my own].''

After hearing Bob Doman speak, and reading his reports, both my husband and I were potential converts. True, every child has different capabilities, and the NACD's viewpoint is a bit extreme. I am not sure that every family would agree with its theories or that every child would thrive in such a program. The point that really struck home with us was the idea of keeping Sophie away from organized groups of children with disabilities. In our minds, as useful as these groups can be, they also serve to emphasize the disability by making it the common bond. Why not simply keep Sophie with children her own age or around those with similar interests? If your child had a broken leg, would you feel obligated to place him or her exclusively with kids with broken legs, or would that be paying unnecessary attention to the problem? As great as some of the well-organized programs for handicapped children are around the country, we suspect they may not be appropriate for our daughter.

This may sound as if we are being snobbish or denying that our child has a problem. Wrong! We're simply denying that the problem needs to be emphasized or exaggerated by placing her exclusively with other disabled children in a large group.

Or it may sound as if we are being too pushy—that maybe we ought to place her where she won't feel intimidated or get left behind. We agree with that point of view. We will not, however, automatically assume that Sophie won't do well, thereby condemning her to classes for children who can't learn or involving her in programs where the expectations are not as high as they should be. I just hope we have a choice.

She's only seven weeks old, so who knows what the future holds? I simply want to give her every opportunity to thrive.

There is more research to be done regarding the NACD program, but already we feel very strongly that Bob Doman is on the right track.

The keynote speaker for the seminar was the mother of an eight-year-old girl with Down Syndrome. Because of the girl's participation in the NACD home program, she was not only a mini-gymnast but also had a reading vocabulary of at least 4,000 words! So much for "your daughter may never learn to read or write"!

We met another set of parents at the seminar whose baby had started to walk at eighteen months with the assistance of the NACD program. This is very early for most babies with Down Syndrome. Many don't walk until the age of two or three, although early intervention and home programs have helped increase the number who do.

We also met a five-year-old girl there who is reading and spelling and speaking beautifully. Many of the negative things we had heard and read were being transformed into myths before our very eyes. Sophie is only a tiny baby, but we are positive she will do as well as, if not better than, each of these children.

Of course we are very vulnerable right now, and our hopes are high that our daughter's future can be assisted in many ways. But this does not mean that we are no longer able to think straight. We will do as much research as necessary in order to accept or reject each therapy presented at the conference. Naturally we want them all to work! We are anxious to believe the doctors and specialists, but we know enough to tread cautiously here. If after our research we feel that some of these therapies may be valuable to Sophie's development, we will pursue them without fail, even if it means breaking the law.

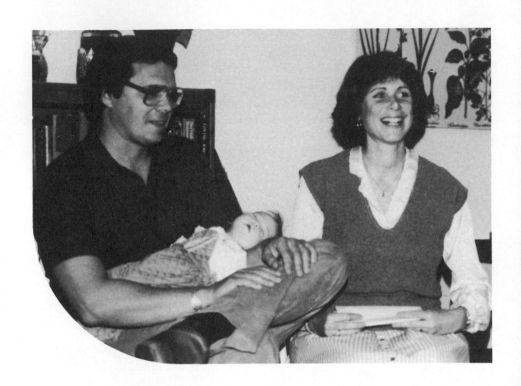

6

Where else can you get whitefish and tears on the same occasion?

November 10. I was thinking about whitefish, food of the Jewish gods, reserved for the happiest of times. I can remember whitefish occasions throughout my entire life: Sunday mornings for a special family treat, family holidays and get-togethers, weddings, celebrations, an addition to a meal when a guest arrived with the oily, pungent package held out as a surprise offering to their delighted hosts.

So for our baby daughter's Naming Ceremony, what food could be more appropriate to serve along with bagels, cream cheese, and salads, than whitefish?

I'd invited the entire family and a few close family friends. I'd asked both sets of grandparents if they'd like to say something during the ceremony. They shyly agreed.

We met with the rabbi to discuss the procedure. We decided upon three Hebrew names for Sophie to honor our relatives. We'd originally tried for four but the rabbi put his foot down! We chose Freydl, after my Grandmother Florence; Yaacova, after my Uncle Jack; and Adina, after Peter's Uncle Adrian.

As you may know, many Jewish male babies are given a ritual circumcision at home by a *mohel*, a rabbi who is trained in this surgical procedure. It is a time of family celebration followed by a party with lots of food.

Over the years another custom, the Naming Cermony, has developed as a way of welcoming girl babies. At this party the baby is given a Hebrew name and, again, everyone gets to eat! The Naming Ceremony is meant to be a joyous occasion, and I wanted Sophie's Naming Ceremony to be no different. I knew some of our friends and relatives had unfounded worries and strange imaginings about how Sophie was doing. The only way to put their minds and hearts at rest was for them to meet her and welcome her to the world. My purpose was also to acknowledge our unique situation and what we had been offering our baby in the way of help and, indeed, what others could do to help. (My secret intention was to show how strong I was and how well I was handling the situation. I did not intend to cry or to show weakness.) I wanted everyone to know my daughter was not a tragedy but a lovable beauty.

Well, all those high-flown intentions lasted until about halfway through the ceremony when the grandparents welcomed Sophie and made their speeches. Somehow I had thought they'd say something light and avoid "the subject." What must I have been thinking? They spoke of acceptance, of love, but also of the sadness of a disability and their desires to help her overcome any obstacles put in her way.

"She will show us new ways to love," said her Grandma Charline.

"I loved her the moment I laid eyes on her. I am so glad she is here," said her Grandpa John.

"We will love Sophie, regardless of her 'chromosomal arrangement.' It is not something like chromosomes that makes us what we are but rather who we are intrinsically," offered her Grandpa Walter.

"I am glad Sophie is in our family. I welcome her and am honored that she was given a Hebrew name for my mother," spoke her Grandma Doris.

There was not a dry eye in the house. It felt so strange to have many of my family members crying together—even strong, able me. It was a horrible and wonderful moment.

Happily, Peter's speech came next. It was funny and affectionate, filled with anecdotes about his Uncle Adrian for whom Sophie was being given a Hebrew name.

I also wrote a speech, fully intending to breeze cheerfully through it. But when my turn came, much to my chagrin I knew I'd never make it through without crying:

"I welcome you all to Sophie's Naming Ceremony. The purposes of this ceremony are to welcome our new baby to the world and to our family and to honor members of her family whom she will never know but who have had an impact on her, nonetheless.

"You are a special hand-picked crowd, chosen because you are closest to us and to our children. Who better than all of you to offer Sophie her first official greeting on planet Earth? In order that she may be properly introduced to each and every one of you, I'm going to ask each of you to introduce yourselves. Please tell her your name, how you are connected to her or to us and also perhaps something you'd like to say to her as part of your hello. Knowing this family, I'll have to suggest that as brilliantly eloquent as we all are, let's leave the major speeches to the rabbi and keep it somewhat brief."

We then went around the room, giving each person present a chance to speak. At the end of the introductions, I continued: "Let's give Sophie and ourselves a round of applause for putting up with each other all this time! For Sophie's Hebrew names Peter and I have chosen three people we have loved and who have had a strong, positive effect on our lives. As you know, a Hebrew name is given for just that reason. It is not simply to find an equivalent for a child's English name but rather a tradition in many Jewish families to honor members of our family no longer here.

"The first of her names is Freydl, in honor of her Great-grandmother Florence, known to all of us as "Gam." Sophie, may you grow to have even a small bit of my grandmother's craziness, compassion, and cockeyed wisdom. She has left you a legacy of Millman madness [Millman was my grandmother's last name] that can only be acquired through that royal bloodline. Gam was one of the hubs in our giant family wheel and now you get to hold on tight for a great ride.

"The second of Sophie's names is Yaacova in honor of her Great-uncle Jack. What a special and sweet man he was. My Uncle Jack was a friend—a warm, thoughtful, and generous person. Sophie, may you acquire his generosity, his genuine interest in and good-heartedness toward all the people he knew. May his uniquely gentle spirit be part of your personality always."

Peter had already spoken about his Uncle Adrian, honored by her third Hebrew name, Adina.

Sophie was bored with all the eloquence and fell asleep right around this part.

"Today I also want to talk about something else. As everyone here knows, Sophie was born with an extra added attraction. Although throughout her life we will try not to dwell on the problems or difficulties that may arise because of her Down Syndrome, or even emphasize the Down Syndrome or discuss it in front of her, I felt it was important to talk about it.

"Sophie is just a tiny baby, and in some ways the label of Down Syndrome becomes bigger than she is. It can sometimes overwhelm someone's response to her, make that person careful or different around us. As her family and friends you have a unique opportunity to treat her not as a baby with a problem but as a sweet, delicious little tot. She may need a bit more of your patience as she grows and a bit more encouragement as well.

"Many of you have asked us if there's anything you can do to help. My answer is a resounding *yes*! You *can* help, and you already have. Here are the things you can continue to do:

1. Maintain your sense of humor at all costs.

2. Keep offering concern and interest. Don't hesitate to ask questions, even nosy ones. We are now ready and strong enough for them! One of the worst things that could happen is that people might tiptoe around the subject. It's not a secret.

3. Tell us anything and everything you hear about that you feel might help or interest us. Everything we've learned that has helped Sophie we've heard about in just that way. There is no "Down Syndrome Central," so we gather information where we can.

4. We've also "learned" some other things that turned out to be untrue. First, let me say that if these things don't ring true with you, they sound totally unreal to us, and we refuse to accept them. For example, on the second day after Sophie was born, a physician in the hospital told us, "Your daughter may never read or write. She may never speak clearly or function above factory-work

mentality." Thankfully, we have since learned that the doctor was referring to children who had been institutionalized many years ago and that his information has no basis in fact today.

"Sophie has no brain injury or damage. We have met many children with Down Syndrome who are walking, talking, reading, writing, and giving their parents a hard time, just like any child. It may simply take a little longer for them to achieve these goals. Our main concern is not that our expectations will exceed her abilities but that her abilities will exceed our expectations. So above all, we need your help to expect and demand the *best* from Sophie. Help us in our endeavor to insist she become excellent at all she attempts to do. She is different from a typical child in that she will need an extra push to get going.

"We already have her involved in the best intellectual and physical stimulation programs we could find, but it is the people surrounding her who will be of the most help in the long run.

"We have a strong intention that Sophie will truly be a star, that she will attend normal school in a normal classroom, that she will read, that she will write. She will run, sing, talk, and tell crummy jokes just like the rest of her family. This is a promise from us to her.

"We have already studied enough and have met enough parents of kids with Down Syndrome to know that, with a lot of work, this is not only possible but will come to be.

"You may think we're expecting too much, that we are being foolish, or that we will be disappointed. Don't worry about that. We just hope we have the energy to keep up with her!

"Some may think it cruel to expect so much from a child in her circumstances; we feel it is cruel *not* to.

"So, to conclude, I'm taking bets from anyone here that every one of our predictions will come true. If you're smart, you'll hold onto your money.

"You can help. You can expect the same as we do. You can assist us. You can put any skepticism or doubt in your pocket or any other convenient place.

"I thank you for being here, and I thank you for helping us keep our promise to Sophie."

✳ ✳ ✳ ✳ ✳

A few days after the ceremony, my mother sent a note saying how much she truly loved the Naming Ceremony. "Where else can you get whitefish and tears on the same occasion?" she wrote. Whitefish and tears. How well my mother summed up the day.

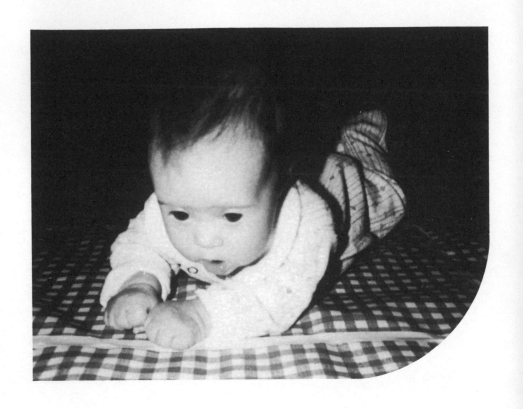

7

We have to do so much work
for so few results

November 11. Sophie is two months old. I keep expecting myself
to snap out of this mood but so far it seems to like my company.
Sometimes I feel it will never go away.

Sophie hardly ever cries. Some parents might be delighted with
such a "good" baby, but I see crying as children's fight for
survival. It's a way of demanding that life come to *them*. She's
also very sleepy and quiet. Maybe this is part of her genetic
problem, or maybe it has something to do with her ear problems.
She lives on antibiotics. I hate giving them to her because they
lower her already low resistance to infection. Still, I'm glad they're
available because at least they do fight the ear infection.

When I really stop to think about it, it seems that I've known
almost nothing but pain, tension, sadness, and the effects of
continually holding back the grief I feel about my child. Sometimes
I even avoid looking at her. The frustration and apathy that
sometimes creep to the surface shock me and fill me with guilt. I
keep waiting for unconditional love to set in. But every morning
when I go to get Sophie out of her crib, I am reminded that
everything is not the way it is supposed to be. With every action I
feel a dull, all-pervasive heaviness, as if someone beat me up for no
reason. I want this all to go away. I feel as if I were in World War
III with explosions, bombs, screams, chaos, and horror that only I
can see. And I have to pretend that I don't feel that way. I can
only communicate fully with other charter members of the "Grief
Club."

Every time someone makes an unwitting comment about my
baby, I just about die. Here is a list of things I never want to hear

again. Although there are more, these are some of the more popular offerings:

1. "Would you have aborted your child, had you known?"

2. "Many people place these babies in foster homes."

3. "People used to institutionalize these babies at birth."

Why does anyone say something so thoughtless? I guess people feel they can be casual with me about the subject because I'm "used to it." But a parent never gets used to being reminded of a child's possible shortcomings or limitations.

About a week ago I went to my first parents' support group offered through Sophie's Infant Stimulation program. About five or six other moms were there, and a social worker led the discussion. Each mother had a child with a different disability. We discussed some of our experiences and shared some helpful suggestions, but no one mentioned feeling depressed. I kept expecting someone to say, "This is so hard for me and for my baby. I'm so unhappy." Either the feelings are too painful or private to bring up, or else I'm the only one who has them! I have to admit that I didn't bring up the subject either. I was secretly afraid that the other moms would think that I didn't love Sophie or that I was crazy or both.

Sometimes I forget that I have a new baby and that she needs the jolly, attentive, fully functioning mother that Max had when he was an infant. My fears and concerns interfere with my ability to show natural affection.

November 16. In spite of my misgivings, I opted to be a "good mother" and took Sophie to the City of Hope research program. The worst part was walking in there. I'm the type that turns the channel to avoid telethons for ill or disabled or abused kids. I can't stand to see little children in dire circumstances. Yet here I was with my own child in a semi-dire circumstance!

The pediatric waiting area was colorful and comfortable, with lots of couches and a TV and toys for the kids. There was even a well-equipped play yard attached to the building. It took everything I had not to burst into tears when I saw that play yard. I kept envisioning terminally ill kids playing on the fancy equipment. I felt such futility. The staff was relentlessly kind and courteous and willing to help. I felt grateful for their compassion, and yet at the same time I didn't *want* their compassion. I mean, who was I to need this kid-glove handling all of a sudden? I kept expecting someone to say, "Look, lady, you'll just have to wait your turn like everybody else!" or "Ma'am, things are tough all over. I've only got one pair of hands, you know." But everyone insisted on being nice. I wondered: is everyone going to be nice to me from now on because they feel sorry for me or my baby, as if being treated "nicely" were somehow my due?

About seven doctors and specialists examined Sophie. There was an ear, nose, and throat specialist; a speech therapist; an occupational therapist; a linguist (who was teaching nonverbal kids to speak with the help of a computer program she had designed); a dentist; a pediatrician; a psychologist. Topping off the exams was a blood test for Sophie's chromosome study. Besides, two nutritionists had to take all of Sophie's measurements twice just to be sure that one of them had not made an error. They bustled around the tiny examining room like Tweedle Dee and Tweedle Dum. Sophie was very good throughout the entire ordeal. She is such a tiny doll, so pretty and good-natured.

After this initial phase, I don't think that I am going to bring her back for the longitudinal study. It's just too demeaning. She doesn't belong to science; she belongs to us. As helpful as some of the data I received was, it was not worth treating her like a specimen.

December 1. The father of the first child with Down Syndrome to start on Dr. H.'s Evoked Potential research program called me today to tell me the incredibly good news. After a full year in the program his daughter's Evoked Potential test was normal! I was filled with cautious joy. The little girl's father said he felt the same way—afraid to get his hopes up, but thrilled nonetheless! Can you blame him? We were both excited on the phone as he related Dr. H.'s enthusiastic reaction to this potentially miraculous milestone. I immediately called Peter at work and made his day! He is so madly in love with Sophie that any positive news at all is as if the heavens

opened up and sent him a personal message. He is confident that
Sophie will surprise all of us with her excellent development. I wish
I had his unendingly optimistic outlook.

December 5. I was just remembering the all-encompassing joy I
experienced when my first child was born. All the exhilaration that
had ever existed in the world was mine. I had done it! A real live
baby boy to love and hold and nurture forever. He looked just like
his papa, was healthy and strapping, and never stopped moving,
crabbing, yelling, or demanding to be fed. There was such an
outpouring of love and excitement from my family and friends.

   This feeling of contentment and simple happiness continued
unabated until Sophie was born. All of a sudden my wellspring
seemed to have dried up. It isn't that I don't love my baby.
Rather, I love her too much. The more affection I feel, the more I
feel my heart break for her. Because the pain comes bounding in
on the heels of my love, it doesn't feel safe to love her so deeply. I
once saw an episode of "Star Trek" in which people had been
tortured and then hypnotically made to forget about it. Every time
the tortured people tried to remember their past, great physical pain
would course through their bodies. For this reason, they chose
detachment from those memories rather than facing that punish-
ment. That's how it is with me—the more I love Sophie, the worse
I feel, so sometimes I become detached rather than closer.

December 12. Sometimes I just can't feel enthusiastic about
Sophie's accomplishments. In her Infant Stimulation class we've
been working on rolling over, head control, and tracking (following
things with her eyes). These are tiring tasks, and I never feel that
I'm doing enough. It's impossible to tell if my work is contributing
to her progress or if she would have made the improvements on her
own.

   But in one area our work *has* produced visible results. Some
days ago we listened to a set of tapes we ordered from the NACD.
One of the suggestions on the tapes was to make a slightly inclined
ramp for your child to practice crawling movements on. As soon as
he heard this, Peter dismantled the double bed in our guest room
downstairs and grabbed the large support board between the

mattresses! With this he went into the garage and made a giant ramp, which he covered with contact paper. He dragged the ramp upstairs and placed his tiny daughter on its surface, pushing her chubby legs and feet down the ramp.

Every evening when he comes home from work, after a marathon game of "tackle" and "stunts" with Max, Peter takes Sophie up to the ramp and, like a drill sergeant, makes her go down the ramp at least three or four times. He's even enlisted Max's help as official cheerleader. I can hear them up there yelling, "Come on, Sophie! No rest for the wicked! Go, go, go!" Sophie crabs and protests the whole time, but Peter is relentless. Knowing Peter, I wouldn't be surprised if it will be the only thing that really works!

December 13. I'm depressed. I sometimes feel we have to do so much work for so few results. But Sophie, at three months old, is making progress in her physical development. Her head is not so wobbly, and her physical strength is improving. She was born with very low muscle tone, a trait typical in infants with Down Syndrome, and is floppy and still very sleepy. Her tracking is improving and she can roll over in both directions, but her vocalization seems to be decreasing rather than increasing. This concerns me.

I often feel so frustrated. I want my daughter to have been born with a healthy body, not one with her chromosomes in a funny pattern. Will I ever be one of those mothers who is thrilled with her child's small successes? I'm always reading about these inspiring mothers of "special children" in popular women's magazines. Will I ever be able to accept the fact that Sophie has an unchangeable, built-in disability and learn to just love her the way she is, problems and all? I don't think I could ever love her problems. Sometimes I just want to scream at her to get her to respond. Always pretending to the world that everything is hunky-dory is exhausting.

We've sent for information about the U-series from Dr. Turkel's office. It's at least worth a closer look.

8

Something has happened in my heart—it's beginning to thaw

December 13. Today there seems to be a ray of hope in my small world. I'm not exactly sure why. Tonight Sophie was laughing and laughing as her papa played "flying baby" with her. She looked great! So cute, so alive and well.

Sophie has begun to push herself up on her hands and look all around wherever she happens to be. She does make a few sounds and laughs and smiles a lot. She can stiffen her legs into a standing position when held up. Her head control is still not what it should be at three months, but I do at least twenty little exercises a day to help improve this—including lifting her up gently by her hands from the floor and sitting her on top of a surface, like a ball or a bolster, to encourage her to hold her head up on her own.

Since Sophie was a week old, Peter has been trying some simple body movement processes on her that he learned in Scientology classes. They really do help to perk her up. When I see her like that, I am filled with laughter myself. I realize that perhaps things aren't so bad after all. She insists on being such a doll that I'm beginning to get over this feeling of peering at her over a fence from a distance. My heart is still heavy, but I believe that I may be able to feel better for longer periods of time.

Talking to Peter last night, I learned that he is just as affected by Sophie's problems but not as overwhelmed by them as I am. Part of the reason is that he works at an exciting job all day and is not the one taking her to doctors and physical therapy and working with her at home on her exercises, constantly reminded of her limitations. For him, life with Sophie is mainly thousands of hugs and kisses as she's handed to him, all sweet-smelling in her clean pj's, and THE RAMP. But I think he also knows that if he were to fall apart—as I seem to have done—there would be no one to run the show. He's been so great! Yet I still feel that motherhood wraps a woman inextricably around the lives of her children in a way that is hard for a father to experience.

We're looking forward to our appointment with the NACD at the end of this month. I want to have a more specific program for Sophie, to eliminate my up-in-the-air feeling about the exercises I am doing with her.

This is the first time I have written in this journal and not cried.

December 16. Things we do with Sophie to help her:

She started physical therapy class at four weeks old. She will soon start speech therapy. According to Dr. H., we should start as early as possible. Every day her papa and I help with her exercises—pulling her up with her hands for head control, helping her scoot by pushing the bottom of her feet, helping her down the ramp, reading to her, showing her many pictures, helping her with visual and mental exercises every day, singing to her, talking to her, getting her to smile and laugh, and working on hand, arm, and leg exercises. How much of each of these activities would be optimum for her I don't know. If we don't keep her on her toes, she'll sleep or doze. But when she is alert and active and laughing, she is very sweet and a beauty.

We took Sophie for her first evaluation at the NACD and got a program for her. Some of it seems like voodoo, and some of it seems helpful. All of it is a mystery. I've never been in this kind of limbo before. Down Syndrome—what an unpredictable condition.

On this visit we saw a nine-year-old girl with Down Syndrome who was very low-functioning. It was also her first visit. She was nonverbal. She snorted and banged the floor with her hand and foot. She crawled. Her mouth and teeth were distorted and chronically open. She paid attention to no one. The look on her mother's face was one of helpless, painful apathy. The mother said she had six other kids and heard about NACD from a friend. How could anyone have gone so long with so little help? Maybe she didn't know there *was* help. Maybe she just couldn't afford it.

What must this child's life be like? What must this *mother's* life be like? I knew that I've made progress when I observed that child and realized that her condition was not inevitable for my daughter. I didn't feel sorrow. I felt a little sad that my daughter was somehow connected to this girl through the same chromosome pattern. But as sure as I know my son will be a star in the sky of life, I know that my sweet baby will rise above her potential inborn physical and mental problems. And I also know that the nine-year-old we met on this visit can improve, now that she has help.

Sophie's new home program from the NACD consists of massaging her body and mouth, rubbing a freezing juice can alternately with a bottle filled with hot water all over her body, exposing her to smells and tastes, spinning with her, tickling her facial nerves, helping her with ramp crawling (we have the ramp!) and half rolls from stomach to side, showing her objects and naming them, mimicking her sounds, practicing her grasp and release, listening to tapes with different sound frequencies—classical music, nursery rhymes, even Gregorian chants! We work on crawling by putting a rolled-up towel under her chest and making her extend her arms to support her weight.

The most complex part of her program is the cross-patterning exercise. Cross-patterning is the moving of a child's body in a crawling motion, alternating opposite hands and feet, just as a healthy baby would crawl. According to Bob Doman at NACD, this proper physical alignment helps mental development as well. Children with disabilities have a tendency to crawl in what Doman refers to as a "homologous pattern," a two-hands, two-feet pattern, instead of using opposite hands and feet. The cross-patterning is an attempt not only to guide an otherwise immobile or improperly moving child into a natural movement, thereby creating a proper developmental schedule, but also to create a normal crawling pattern once the child does move on his or her own. For Sophie, this exercise requires at least two people to move her arms, legs, and head for five minutes, three times a day. We'll see if all of this does any good.

✳ ✳ ✳ ✳ ✳

I've started to gauge people by how I feel they would treat my daughter now or in the future.

It's weird to experience the first-time reactions of some of the people who have known about Sophie's Down Syndrome *before* they have met her. One such couple looked at her in the stroller with strange expressions of concern and pity. Too bad. She is not an object of pity at all! She is a sweet "chubbette" who is doing remarkably well. (*I'm* the one who needs the pity!)

December 20. Something has happened in my heart—it's beginning to thaw. Maybe the reason is that we now have a program that will help Sophie, and I see that we're on the right course. It's been a very long three and a half months. I still cry almost every day. But Sophie is becoming more real to me. She says "goo" and "oo-eh." I'm liking her.

Both Peter and I are starting to understand some of the difficulties of Sophie's situation after seeing an episode of "The Fall Guy" on TV. The show starred a young boy with Down Syndrome. Although we were thrilled that he could read beautifully, could speak clearly, and was physically adept, we both saw, for the first time, that even with all these exciting accomplishments, the boy was still mentally delayed. We are only beginning to face that difficult, heartbreaking possibility for our Sophie. I can tell this is particularly hard for my husband. But I'm coming out of my gloom a little, so maybe I can help *him*!

Sochie (one of her nicknames) likes her NACD program, but finding time enough to do all of it is hard. Since it takes two people to do the cross-patterning exercises, I put an ad in the local paper for volunteers to help:

> Volunteers needed in my home to help
> our baby with "patterning" exercises,
> to aid in her delayed development.
> Will choose a time convenient to your
> schedule. Please call Jolie with any
> questions. Thank you!

I included my phone number so people could reach me if they were interested. I really thought the ad would be a waste of money. I doubted that anyone would want to volunteer for this sort of thing. Guess what? So far *six* people have called. From what I could gather from our brief phone conversations, they are all different and interesting.

In everything I do regarding Sophie's disabilities, I feel an ache— regret, disappointment, something—even when good things are happening, like people volunteering to help. I never would have had the opportunity to meet them if it weren't for Sophie. So in a way being Sophie's mother is opening up an avenue I never would have traveled. But it's still a nightmare. I continue to fantasize that she's well and healthy and sparkling, but, even more amazingly, sometimes I now see her as herself.

I still can't handle being alone in the car. That's when I'm nowhere: there are no distractions, just the road and my thoughts.

Sometimes I feel the only way to rid my mind of sad thoughts is to write them down. These next thoughts fill me with guilt, but I can't deny them. I am going to write a memorial service for the daughter I "lost." I feel bad even having these thoughts, but they exist.

I think my expectations for my own children were formed as soon as I started playing with dolls. This is especially true about a daughter. All my dolls were baby girls. I dressed them in feminine clothes, assigned them specific attributes such as beauty and brilliance, and generally demanded that they conform to my mold of perfection. I knew with absolute certainty that this is what it would be like to have a *real* baby. And I also knew a daughter would grow up to be as neat as a Barbie doll, perhaps a glamorous career woman or a brilliant surgeon.

So for me it's as if a death occurred for which there was no funeral and no socially prescribed behavior. It was the death of my expectations, my imagined future, and the imagined future of my daughter. For nine months I fantasized about this child, our family, how we would all be. I still do; only the future is filled with mystery now. I face either an unknown or an unwillingness on my part to know. I fantasized my daughter with freckles, of course, and with a reddish tint in her hair. And devilish and talkative and demanding. And smart. So smart you would be taken aback by her precociousness. This daughter would be "one of the girls" who would shop with me for beautiful clothes for her dates and who would go to lunch with me and my mother and aunt and sister and cousin and gossip and laugh and joke. Don't tell me, "Well, Sophie may be able to do those things!" in a bright and cheery voice. How does the term "mental retardation" sound to you? Right now it seems to take over so much of my hope.

This is not to say that Sophie is not well-loved and that she could not have been born into a family that could adore her more. That is not my point. All that is always true. But there are also other truths, and sometimes they bombard me more harshly than the sweet ones do.

✳ ✳ ✳ ✳ ✳

Either just before or while I was newly pregnant with Sophie, I had a very vivid dream. So vivid in fact that I mentioned it to my husband in the morning.

I dreamed I had a child with Down Syndrome. In the dream I was at an elegant party—a fundraising event—with well-dressed people. Also present were children with Down Syndrome. Their parents were holding champagne glasses. The furnishings were sparse and the floors were polished wood. We were at the home of a foundation located in a charming Spanish-style building, pink on the outside with red brick tiles on the roof and a brown wood balcony encircling the second story. In front was a small parking lot, and there was another in a leaf-filled area. The building was surrounded by eucalyptus trees. It was cold outside, as in the fall. I remember clearly that everyone was friendly and content and proud of this event, and I awoke with a feeling of peace and comfort. My thought in the dream was it's okay to have a child with Down Syndrome; it's really not a tragedy. I remember thinking as I awoke that it was an odd thought to have. This dream was different from the regular confused goings-on in most dreams; it was very clear, like a message from myself.

9

Sometimes life deals you
a wild card or two

December 28. I know I am not the first parent to suffer the dilemma of how to announce the birth of a child born with exceptionalities. When Max was born, I sent out a joyous typewritten announcement printed on colorful paper, which described the long labor and delivery and the height, weight, and feistiness of our new son.

When Sophie was born, I knew I had to tell close friends and relatives the whole story. But I also felt she merited the same kind of joyful birth announcement. How to do both of these things in one announcement was a challenge I mulled over for many days. Finally the answer came to me: I would send a lighthearted birth announcement bragging about our daughter to friends, acquaintances, work associates, and everyone else we knew. Then, a while later, I would send out my regular newsletter describing the whole situation. The newsletter would go only to people close to us who I felt would be a part of Sophie's life and would want to know about her problems, her programs, and her progress.

This is Sophie's birth announcement:

QUEEN SOPHIE ARRIVES IN A BLAZE OF GLORY!

Yes, friends and family, Ms. Sophie Kanat-Alexander flew into the world on September 11, 1984, weighing a hefty 8 pounds 7 ounces and measuring 21 inches in length. Unlike her brother who took approximately thirty-six hours to make his entrance, La Sophie took only three action-packed hours to debut at Westlake Hospital in the very trendy Family Birthing Center. It took only a few days for her closet to be filled to the brim with pink, pink, pink, and more pink!

Of course the color looks spectacular on her and puts a glow into her chubby cheeks.

If you were hoping that with the arrival of Madame Sophie the newsletters would stop — you couldn't be further from the truth! I'm sure you'll all be delighted to know that they will most probably be at least twice as long! More ground to cover and twice as much bragging to be done now that we have two of the most spectacular children in the universe.

Love,
Peter, Jolie, Max and Sophie!

And this is a portion of the newsletter that followed about a month and a half later:

THE MAX AND SOPHIE REPORT

Well, I'm sitting here with Max and Sophie, listening to "Yentl" on the stereo. It's the first night of Chanukah. Max is playing with his beloved new Tinkertoys. Sophie just rolled over and is staring intently at her new wind-up merry-go-round toy. Sounds pretty sweet, doesn't it? At least they're both quiet for a few precious moments.

Max is, at long last, adjusting to the fact that his kingdom is altered forever with the entrance of the Queen. He is growing into a handsome, smart, funny, stubborn, relentlessly inquisitive boy. He truly loves his new sister, but hates us for bringing her home! He is making new friends on the block and has lots of buddies at preschool. He's like a minimacho guy. It's so strange to see him sprout away from his boyhood and leap into the world of discussions of the moon, how trees grow, and "Why don't we have Christmas lights on our house?" It's even more interesting trying to figure out how to answer him. He might start piano lessons soon too! He seems to have an endless interest in records, singing, and instruments of all kinds. He also loves to build anything and wants to know how everything is made. Even though he's devilish, he is a shining light in our lives.

We have made the adjustment to having two kids pretty easily, mainly because we were already parents. Of course, with Sophie's birth came an unexpected surprise—which brings us to the next paragraph.

As you may know, Sophie was born with Down Syndrome. At three months old, she is doing very well. She is attending a physical therapy class and will soon be involved in a program in our home, so that both her mama and papa can participate. Due to everyone's help, an early diagnosis, and lots of work on our part, we are determined that she will do as well as is humanly possible. This is not exactly the kind of thing that we had envisioned writing to you about in our semiannual letter, but sometimes life deals you a wild card or two. Sophie is cute as a bug and is very active. She has gained about five pounds and has grown two and a half inches! She is in love with the bells hanging in her playpen.

More than at any other time in our lives, we need the support of our friends and family, and you have come through! I know it sounds corny, but we have learned how nice you bums can be. So, keep it up!

So, we hope that all is well with all of you. This has been an— uh—interesting year, filled with events that "alter and illuminate our time." Mostly alter.

As my sainted mother would say, "Life is mysterious. Don't take it serious."

Love,
Peter, Jolie, Max, and Sophie

✳ ✳ ✳ ✳ ✳

I asked parents in a similar situation how they handled their birth announcements. Each set of parents of a baby with disabilities had their own way of sharing their child's entrance to the world. My friends Jay and JoAnn combined an announcement with a newsletter and managed to not only educate their friends and family but also move them deeply:

Dear friends and relatives,

Happy Holidays! We hope everyone had a healthy and successful year. We had an extremely busy and eventful one. The most exciting and significant event was the birth of our beautiful daughter, Jaclyn, on May 15. She started out a mere 5 lbs. 12 oz. and 18 inches and has now (at seven months) made it to 12½ lbs. and 23½ inches. She has brought us much happiness and joy. She has been such a happy and good baby that we have been able to take her with us almost anywhere. In fact, within her first month she was attending school with JoAnn at UCLA.

As most of you already know, she has also brought us tears. Several hours after our beautiful baby girl was born the doctors informed us that she had Down Syndrome. One week later this was confirmed through a blood test which looks at her genetic material. All normal cells have forty-six chromosomes which control all functioning. Jackie has forty-seven. This condition is not reversible and it is the most common chromosomal birth defect. No one yet knows the cause of this. We have been assured that it is not caused by anything that we did or did not do. In a very small percentage of cases the mother or father is a carrier. This, however, is not true in our case. This birth defect occurs at conception when the fertilized egg first divides, and babies are born with it in 1 out of 700 births. The chances of us having other normal children are still very high and when the right time comes, we will try again.

The symptoms of Down Syndrome are many. They include characteristic facial features, various anthropometric changes, possible medical problems, and mental and physical delay—the degree of which can only be known as time passes. If Jackie's first seven months are any indication of her future, she will be one of the lucky ones. She has been developing wonderfully in all areas. To help her along, she goes to school twice a week with JoAnn to work on physical development and to teach JoAnn how to provide the right stimulation at home. They also go to a Mommy and Me class once a week with normal kids. In January they will start speech therapy every Friday. In addition to these programs we are researching three medical programs and one physical regimen—none of which are generally accepted by the medical establishment or the FDA.

The most frustrating thing about Down Syndrome is that there is no "right" way to help Jackie reach her potential. It is all more or less controversial and we are basically left on our own to decide what will or will not be harmful or beneficial. The tremendous bright spot is that the parent community is very supportive and we have met many very nice people and have lots of great friends who have the same problems and experiences as we do.

Many of our relatives and friends have asked what they can do to help. The absolute most important thing you can do is to accept Jackie into your hearts and treat her as you would any other child. She is extremely lovable and makes us very, very happy.

We all hope that your year was special and that the upcoming years are healthy, happy, and prosperous.

Happy holidays and happy New Year,
Jay, Jackie, and JoAnn

Another couple, the Boyajians, sent this simple and touching announcement:

Now

we

are

three

Though in some ways Brandon is less than perfect, God's miraculous way of compensating should be comfort and joy for us all. God has chosen us to be the parents of this "special" boy. We ask the love, support and prayers of our family and friends to help us raise Brandon to his highest potential.

Brandon Jon

August 12, 1984

7 lbs., 6 oz.

20 inches

Brad and Glenda Boyajian

✳ ✳ ✳ ✳ ✳

Many parents mentioned nothing in their announcements, feeling the announcement should just be a simple statement to the world of the birth of their baby.

Each family has to do what feels best. I found from my own experience that most people in your life want to know about your child's progress and setbacks, and some people don't ever need to know, depending upon how close or distant the relationship is.

I also found that if you share what's in your heart, the world reaches out to you. This is truly a chance for the absolute best in people to come out and shine. It's also their chance to be tacky and unintentionally thoughtless. I've learned to brace myself for every type of response imaginable.

10

I had to give that doll away

December 30. Two days ago I was in the local toy store to return
some duplicate gifts Sophie had received for the holidays. There on
the counter were two of the elusive Cabbage Patch dolls so desired
by thousands. Instead of buying Sophie some new things, I bought
one of the dolls in exchange for the gifts. The price of the doll was
outrageous. My spur-of-the-moment justification was that I bought
the Cabbage Patch doll for Sophie, who is just three and a half
months old.

Just as background: I had been longing secretly for an adorable
red-haired, blue-eyed Cabbage Patch doll and couldn't figure out
why, since I wasn't really into dolls at all. I guess I know why now;
I wanted a baby with no problems. I wanted a perfect baby. If I
bought the doll, I could at least look at her and fantasize.

I brought the doll home, but for two days I couldn't bring myself
to open up the box and take her out. Max kept asking me,
"Mommy, when are you going to take the Cabbage Patch doll out
of her box so we can play with her?" I felt foolish. I didn't
understand why I couldn't just open the box. I had even opened it
a little to peek at the name on the "birth certificate": Gayla
Gaylene.

Finally I decided to accept the fact that I bought her for myself,
not for my daughter. I had been hoping I could think of someone
to give her to, because Sophie was obviously too young to play with
the doll and it was so ridiculously expensive. I could save the doll
for a couple of years for her but by that time she'd probably
demand a brand-new doll anyway.

I opened up the box and put the doll on the couch. She was
really cute. My sister, Jaime, came over to show us her new car
and I took Gayla Gaylene along for a ride. Before I left I took one

of Sophie's blankets to cover the doll so she wouldn't get wet from the rain. Peter saw me take the blanket and gave me a strange look. I knew the jig was up; I knew my husband knew that this was a flaky deal. During the ride with Jaime I asked her if she would like to take the doll home. She also looked at me as if I were nuts—and refused. I told her she could take it until I found a new home for her. I did not want that doll in my house! She said no. We laughed about it.

After that I needed to do some grocery shopping. And I *had* to find someone who was perfect for that doll. Actually, it didn't really matter *who* I found—I just felt guilty having the doll. Sure enough, the woman checking out my groceries started talking about how hard it was to find a Cabbage Patch doll. I told her I had one that really should belong to about a three-year-old child. She said her neighbor had been looking for one for her three-year-old daughter but either couldn't find one or couldn't afford one. She asked how much I would sell it for. Although earlier that day I'd been thinking of giving it away, I said twenty-five dollars. She said, "Sold!" I rushed home, asked Peter to put the groceries away, and tore back to the store to give her the doll. What a relief.

I'm still unhappy about the entire, strange incident but I felt so guilty about having that doll. I really wanted her, and I want her still. What I really want is for my Sophie to be perfect, like the doll. I had to give that doll away because I have to give those *ideas* away.

Would having another baby generate the same feelings of guilt, making me feel that I was trying to "replace" Sophie? Maybe so. But I wouldn't be able to give that baby away to a check-out woman in the supermarket. Even if she were to offer me twenty-five dollars!

December 31. I've had a sore throat for three months. Sometimes I've coughed all night, and at other times I've had trouble swallowing. At one point it turned into an ear infection. I'm always thirsty. Right now the infection has landed on the left side of my throat. There's no medical treatment for this because I know it's caused by suppressed grief—by "swallowing" my grief, my thoughts, or my responses. They've accumulated there and turned into an ache that's stubborn and tenacious and taunting.

There are, however, whole long moments when I'm just fine, when Sophie is just my baby, when I kiss her chubby cheeks and work with her on her program and sing to her. She is a wide-eyed, urchin-faced tot. Her eyes are beautiful. Her skin is pink and ivory. She is about twenty-four inches long and weighs twelve-and-a-half pounds; she's tiny but growing very well. Her hair is very dark with hints of auburn, and there's lots of it. Right now she is supposed to be sleeping—it's 10:30 P.M.—but she just woke up and is chewing her thumb and propping herself up on her hands to look all around. She is very quiet, and this kills me. I want her to be a blabbermouth, but I suppose I should give her a little more time!

I'm starting a sign language class in February, speech therapy for her, and a special speech class for infants at a local university. God forbid my daughter shouldn't be able to communicate in any way possible the very minute she becomes able to!

The little Soche (another nickname—rhymes with "coach") refuses to take a bottle, so I've never been away from her for more than four hours at a time—usually not for more than two hours. In a way this is good, because it keeps me connected to her. Sometimes I feel I might just run away forever if I didn't have to be home to feed her.

It occurs to me that now is probably one of the very best times of Sophie's life and of our life with her. Because she is a tiny baby there are few indications of delay and few physical characteristics to show Down Syndrome. And I am wasting this potentially happy time on grief and worry and regret.

More and more often, though, I feel flickers of really noticing who she is.

It's my fantasy life that is very affected. For example, every time I look closely at her I suppress thoughts I would normally be having—even though she's only three and a half months old. Like, "What career will you choose?" "What college will you be attending?" "Whom will you marry?" This happens a dozen times a day. It overloads my circuits just turning these thoughts off.

Most times we have so much fresh energy and hope for Sophie. Yet sometimes I watch myself at a distance—having this hope and at the same time *knowing* our energy and enthusiasm may well dissipate over time as we see what is impossible to believe or accept: mental retardation. I think, although we've never said this out loud to one another, that Peter and I both believe that Sophie will be the first child with Down Syndrome ever to escape retardation of any kind. At the same time, I've accepted the fact that she will not escape this. She wants to nurse, so my battling thoughts will have to wait until later.

January 1. My mom bought me a subscription to a magazine called *Exceptional Parent.* After reading it cover to cover, I discovered something amazing: compared to the disabilities and medical problems faced by the kids described in that magazine, Down Syndrome is like a vacation in Tahiti! What, no surgery? No spastic movements or seizures? No drooling or constant vomiting? Why, there wasn't even one measly article on a kid with Down Syndrome in the entire magazine! Down Syndrome doesn't even rate in the "Who's Worse?" contest.

I sometimes play a "Who's Worse?" contest with myself when I'm in Sophie's Infant Stimulation class or at a children's hospital or at the NACD. I observe kids with severe disabilities—brain damage, failure to thrive, cerebral palsy—and I say to myself about each one, "Let's see, yes, he or she is definitely worse." As if this strange form of competitive thinking makes my daughter less "exceptional" in some way. My intention is not to be cruel. There's an unwanted, unspoken contest of awfulness going on. Sophie never wins! She's always in the best shape of them all. My mother has a saying: "In order to appear thin, hang out with fatties." Sophie always seems so alert around those kids! I think other moms make the same observations about their impaired children, regardless of the disability. For me, this way of thinking is a protective mind game. Sometimes I feel totally unworthy of sympathy or help. Down Syndrome is a picnic compared with these other disabilities! Funny how my whole point of view can change from one moment to the next.

The fact that Sophie is very, very cute right now doesn't keep away my thoughts of how she may look later. But she is truly pretty and bright and alert. She smiles in her sleep. She laughs all the time. She is perfectly formed. Her "Down's" nose looks just like a button baby nose. Her papa adores her. He is kissing her tummy right now and she is laughing, laughing, laughing! Sometimes I feel that if it weren't for my husband I couldn't be a normally functioning person right now. He makes everything better with his sense of humor and absolutely positive attitude.

January 2. Today Sophie's first volunteer came to help with cross-patterning. She is a beautiful girl, fifteen years old, who "just wants to help." Where do these people *come* from? I taught her the cross-patterning exercise, and she really did help.

I also talked to a woman in Oregon today about cell therapy. I still need to do more research. She told me that her fifteen-month-old son with Down Syndrome was not yet creeping on all fours, just crawling on his tummy. I think Sophie will be creeping at a normal age. She's already "combat crawling" a little bit because of the NACD's and Peter's exercise programs. "Combat crawling" is a term used to describe the crawling a baby does by pulling herself along, flat on her tummy, with elbows and arms and some legwork, instead of up on all fours. Her combat crawling is not a cross-pattern, but at least she's moving! She can crawl mostly on her own power down Peter's homemade ramp, and the cross-patterning seems to increase her enthusiasm for the real thing! So we'll see. She's almost four months old and making more sounds more often. I'm going to get her ears checked again. I'm concerned that she's never had a startle reflex to loud sounds.

January 4. A private physical therapist came to the house yesterday because Infant Stimulation is closed for Christmas vacation through New Year's Day. When the physical therapist was working with her, Sophie crawled halfway across the mat all by herself! It was a breathtaking moment for me and surprised the physical therapist as well. We've been doing the cross-patterning for about one and a half weeks and I know that it is helping very much.

Tonight I was looking at her sleeping in my arms, and she was so pretty. For some reason that was upsetting. I'd be upset if she weren't pretty, and I'm upset that she is pretty. Don't ask me why. I can hardly explain it to myself.

Yesterday I had two friends over for lunch in honor of one of their birthdays. As one friend watched me holding Sophie, she exclaimed, "Oh, her head's so little! How cute!" I almost died. Then later she said, "You know, I got your newsletter and I really think it's great how you've *accepted it* and all." I knew her intentions were good, but something about her tone annoyed me. I said "Well, you know, it's like if a dog came up to you and lifted a leg on your jeans—you could pretend it hadn't happened. Or you could face the situation and handle the problem. It's not really a question of acceptance; it's a question of reality." I felt like snapping at her and I did. At least it kept me from telling her not to be a jerk and thereby ruining our friendship. But somehow I think the friendship may be on the way out anyway.

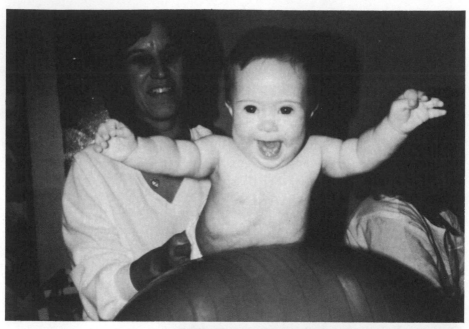

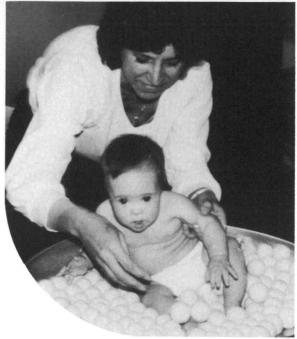

11

We are a whole family,
not just a Sophie family

January 5. Max has an imaginary brother. He mentioned him for
the first time a couple of days ago. Today we asked Max some
questions about him. His name is Dinky. He's taller than Max.
They play together. Max said he bought Dinky a bed. Peter was
taking Max to a college basketball game today, so I asked Max if
Dinky was going with him. He said no. When he came back many
hours later I asked him again (just checking) if Dinky was at the
game. He said, "No, he's upstairs sleeping." Max discusses Dinky
with total seriousness, not laughing or joking at all. There's no
doubt in Max's mind that Dinky exists, so there's nothing to laugh
about, I guess.

We are trying to even the balance of attention shown to our kids,
but it's hard. I've scheduled Sophie's volunteers during the day
when Max is at preschool so we can spend as much time as possible
with Max when Peter is home. Since Sophie's sleeping schedule is
not yet firmly established, Max goes to sleep much earlier than
Sophie (the party girl), so Peter spends time with her *after* Max goes
to bed. We're trying not to make Sophie's disabilities seem "neat"
just because she gets a lot of attention for them. I can just picture
Max creating illnesses or accidents to get that kind of attention. Is
he doing that with Dinky?

We are a whole family, not just a Sophie family. If spending a
little more time with Max means that Sofe (another nickname)
doesn't get to continue with some part of her program, it's a
necessary compromise. But we feel torn sometimes.

＊ ＊ ＊ ＊ ＊

Tonight two pageants were on TV. One was for "Mother/
Daughter" pairs of 1985. The other was "Miss Teenage America."

Even though I have never put much store in beauty contests, I was struck with how fundamental perfect smiles and predictability are to acceptance and popularity. Knowing that Sophie and I won't be that picture-perfect mother/daughter pair of 1998 hurts, even though it's a contest I'd never enter anyway! Perhaps because I feel that as a mother and daughter Sophie and I may be different from what's expected, it is harder for me to enjoy all the glitz and glitter of these events. That a contest like "Miss Teenage America" would be ruled out for my daughter makes me resent the whole thing. Before now I wouldn't have given it a second thought.

January 7. You know that old saying, "God never gives you more than you can handle"? Who in the world made that up? Let me understand just what it implies: God has chosen you, Jolie Kanat, to have a child with Down Syndrome because you are such a strong, grand, and glorious person that *you* can handle it! If you couldn't handle it, it would never have happened. If you had been blessed with instability, personality problems, a crummy marriage, and a rotten family, God wouldn't have bestowed this child upon you. But, lucky you, you qualify for a free lesson in adversity.

Look, God, how about a small fire, a hurricane, or a serious case of chicken pox instead? Something that goes away. Something I can protect my child from.

January 8. I have been trying to find an analogy for the conflicting feelings I have about loving my little daughter. Imagine you are in a wild jungle so thick and high you have to cut and chop your way with a machete. At your feet are snakes and bugs that frighten you and distract you from your task. You have actually been promised a sightseeing, nature, and bird-watching trip by the travel agent who set this up. Obviously, there are certain priorities that need attending to before you can look up to notice the fine points of a rare bird or the simple beauty of an exotic tropical flower. In fact, you are so busy handling the obstructions and threats in your path that you never do have the chance to enjoy your surroundings. By the time you create a small cleared-away resting area, you are too exhausted and distracted to notice any birds or flowers. You gobble down your lunch and continue on through the untamed tropics, cursing the travel agent and planning how to get your money back from that smooth-talking creep.

What I'm trying to explain is my feeling of frustration at trying to simply love a child who brings such difficulty and effort and uncertain hopes. It's hard to peek through all the trouble to see a tiny, sweet, lovable baby there.

January 9. Today was quite a full day for Sofe. While Max was at preschool I took her to Infant Stimulation. Then we went home for two or three hours of NACD program activities, then the physical therapist came to visit and evaluate Sophie, and then her volunteer came for cross-patterning. It was crazy scheduling on my part, and I thought Sophie would surely be exhausted from all the goings-on. I know I was! But just the opposite occurred. She was bright-eyed and bushy-tailed. That's when I realized what I already knew but hadn't wanted to face: more is better. I could work with her seven hours a day and she'd be delighted. She'd probably be doing better, but of course, I'd be going nuts. It almost seems as if the only times Sophie is fully alive and alert is when we're working with her. She can last on her own for a couple of hours in the evening before sputtering out. Those are my most rewarding times because she looks so beautiful and vital. (And of course, her papa is home to help!)

Unless there's a cheerleading section, she goes to sleep, chews on her hand, or puts her head down and looks quietly at a toy. Often when I put her in her crib while I do some chore, she's absolutely quiet. I walk back in to her room, thinking she must be asleep. Instead I see her looking quietly at her mobile or a doll, and I have an eerie feeling. Times like those make my stomach sink, and I think, I should be doing something with this tot right now. I sense that the moments I spend doing something else are times her life is dwindling or remaining static—that she won't improve or thrive on her own. In some ways this makes me feel needed, and in others it makes me feel desperate.

Tonight I had a stray, unconnected thought as I was walking into the supermarket: I am very small. I am small and little and I don't belong here.

January 14. Right now I feel moderately happy again. I got some counseling from a Scientology counselor and I had a realization: I am in charge of how long this mourning period continues. I laughed when I realized that. And you know something? Sophie is doing much better too. She is stronger, more alert, more awake, funnier and more responsive. Maybe that's just in my mind, but I know there's a correlation between how I'm feeling and how she's feeling. It makes sense, since we're around each other so much.

The amount Sophie babbles has decreased, and she's been congested for a month or so, so I took her to the ear, nose, and throat specialist today. Flat tympanogram. More fluid. More antibiotics. During my monthly phone reports to Dr. H., she keeps saying Sophie's going to need tubes. I hope not. If I can just keep her sinuses cleared up!

Because the doctor's appointment lasted so long and I then had to stop at the pharmacy for a refill of Sophie's Vitamin B_6 and magnesium, I didn't pick up Max from preschool until 5:30! That's the latest he's ever been there. I felt terrible. He seemed just fine, but I felt frustrated that I didn't have close relatives nearby who could pick him up when something like this happens.

We are trying so hard not to make Max a casualty of the Down Syndrome syndrome. The other day he asked us, "When is Sophie's Down Syndrome going to be over?" The question just kind of hung in the air for awhile. Then I answered, "Well, sweetie, she's always going to have it. It's just something she was born with." He seemed to understand a little.

January 17. Right now I hate my daughter. I got so mad when for the third or fourth time in a row, she spit out her vitamins and refused to take them! I hate her. I hate her vitamins. I hate her life. I hate my life. I hate that she was born. I hate motherhood. I hate crying. I hate my friend for having a healthy baby girl yesterday. I hate that everything went right for her and everything went badly for me. I hate everything. Why isn't my daughter normal? I hate whoever the fool was who invented the concept of fairness.

I talked in the Infant Stimulation parents' group about my feelings today. Usually it's not like me to make myself so vulnerable, but this time I did get some helpful responses. One mom said, "Look, *any* kid can be a problem. What kid ever fulfills a parent's every dream?"

In a way she had a point. But that's not really very applicable here, because sometimes I feel I have *no* dreams for Sophie. That's really an empty and dark and quiet feeling. I can't be cheer-led into thinking there are dreams to be had. This is not exactly pessimism—it just seems like the truth. But then again, I can always think of the kids with much more severe disabilities and realize that, yes, by comparison, there *are* dreams to be had. *Hopes* may be a little more accurate. Hopes for intelligence, hopes for full physical function. But these are so spare, so devoid of the stuff of life. Am I so selfish to want everything to be perfect with my child? Isn't this how any normal mother feels? Aren't all mothers crazy on the subjects of the health and intelligence and futures of their children? I feel guilty when I realize that what I'm feeling is not just concern for Sophie, but concern and despair for myself—for my crooked future, for my pretend existence in the meantime.

If one more person tells me, "God has a purpose for Sophie," or "God had a plan for you," or "God loves you," I'm tempted to help straighten that person out in a big way. If it's so "godly" to have a baby with Down Syndrome, then why aren't these people disappointed that they don't have one of their own? I'm still waiting for the halo to appear on my saintly head.

The other day my friend JoAnn said to me that I'm pursuing a lot of activities—maybe too many. Infant Stimulation two days a week, NACD about two hours a day, speech on Fridays, physical therapy at home (I'm planning to start that once a week), the City of Hope parents' group, the volunteers every day, and then, of course, Max's preschool, pre-reading and math classes, and soon piano lessons. And sign language classes. You know, I think I ought to do something for myself. A lot of this *is* for myself, but it's not very luxurious. What could I do? A job? That would be pretty neat. But it's too soon for that. What else? I'd love to work. I'd love to wean Sophie, hire someone to watch her and Max, and go to work part time. It doesn't sound that complicated, does it? But it's too soon.

In the meantime, Dinky is sleeping in the downstairs bathroom.

January 18. I feel as if PMS has taken over my life, but in truth, because of pregnancy and nursing, I haven't had a period in over a year! I feel so crabby today that I think the only excuse possible is that my period's near. A new volunteer for cross-patterning came today. She is a single mother who has adopted three special-needs kids—one was abused in infancy, one is hydrocephalic, and one is learning-disabled and emotionally disturbed. She works full time and wants to help Sophie during her lunch hour! She's a very interesting woman. At least I'm not bored. Neither is she, I would imagine.

My little son is the shining light in my life. He fills me with joy. He takes away my glumness with his fast talking and sweet sense of humor. He makes me laugh a lot. He is adjusting very well now to being dethroned. He calls Sophie "Tiny True" and "Beautiful B." They beam when they see each other. We were in a restaurant the other day waiting to be seated, when he pointed up toward the wall and said, "Mommy, look! A macaroni motor home!" I looked and looked and couldn't figure out what he could be referring to. Then I noticed a picture of a San Francisco cable car. Aha! Rice-a-roni commercials have a cable car. He confused that with macaroni. It took a while, but I figured out that to him a cable car is a "Macaroni motor home." That boy makes me laugh!

January 20. Sophie is four and a half months old.

Guess what? It really *was* PMS. I'm so thrilled that my crabbiness was due to hormonal havoc and not creeping insanity. I feel much better.

Sophie is starting to scoot a lot. She's grabbing at her toys. She semi-scoots over to get a favorite plaything. She is the only kid in her Infant Stimulation class who exhibits scooting ability, and some of the kids are nearly a year old. At four months, her muscle tone is improving. She doesn't hold her head perfectly straight but nearly so, and there's almost no wobble. She is getting strong and much more able. She laughs about a thousand times a day. She always laughs when I play a game with her called "Bite Your Mommy's Nose!" In her glee and delight, her cute face wrinkles up and her chubby fists come together.

A mother in the Infant Stimulation parents' support group adopted a "high-risk" infant a few months ago. The baby, who was premature with a brain hemorrhage at birth, is a high risk for neurological disorders—mental retardation or cerebral palsy—and the accompanying difficulties. Apparently this woman was having an impossible time conceiving and the birth parents did not even want this child to *live*. The adoptive mother was the baby's neonatal nurse, and she fell in love with him. Four weeks after the adoption she got pregnant! Her baby is due in May. The babies will be thirteen months apart.

Another mother in the class is in the process of trying to adopt a four-week-old baby with Down Syndrome for whom she is now a foster mother. She also has other foster children.

Then there's Sophie's volunteer with the three adopted special-needs kids.

Seeing these women raises an internal conflict: I did not *choose* to have a baby with a disorder—how could *they*? Even though we all have children with similar problems, our points of view must really diverge. The moms who gave birth to these babies are thinking "Why me? Why my baby?" On the other hand, the moms who chose these kids are *choosing* an incredible challenge. These mothers have my admiration, but they also have my wonder. How could they have jumped into this with their eyes wide open?

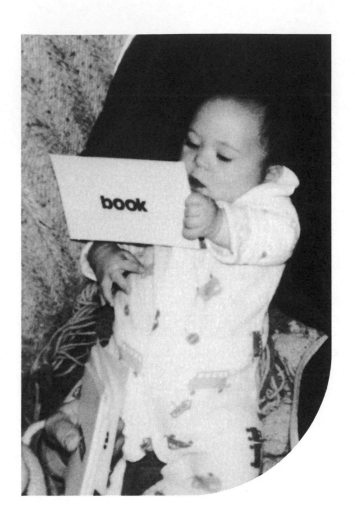

12

I do have dreams for Sophie

January 21. I received the information on cell therapy that I had
sent for. It sounds promising. Its foremost advocate, Dr. Schmid,
is no flake, but to date the treatment is not accepted in the United
States. Travel to Germany and accommodations and the cells
themselves are, of course, all expensive. The treatment is considered unorthodox, but many parents rave over its results with their
kids. I'd like to talk to some dissatisfied customers to hear their
points of view too.

I've observed a phenomenon. Many mothers of kids with Down
Syndrome are unable to see any physical or mental problems in
their own children. One mother recently said to me, "The geneticist just couldn't tell if my baby was Downs. I can't see any
features myself." Observing this child from a more objective point
of view, I noticed that his eyes were crossed and very puffy and his
head size was a bit distorted and, in short, he didn't look that great
to me.

Another mother had called me when Sophie was about two
weeks old, offering to bring her two-and-a-half-year-old son with
Down Syndrome to my home so I could see how cute he was. I
was terrified to see an older child at that very tender time in my life,
and I made an excuse so she wouldn't come. Well, just last week
this same mother said she had a book for me and wanted to bring it
to my house. She also brought her son, who, it turned out, truly
was cute. But, at almost three years old, he was very small and
exhibited some obvious mental delay. He probably functioned
somewhere around the eighteen-month level. Seeing this cute little
guy was comforting in some ways, but I suspect that would not
have been the case four months ago. The woman's intentions,

however, were so good that I really harbor only positive feelings toward her.

These are examples of how one-sided a mother's vision of her child can be. I think most mothers are that way; they extol their children's virtues, and you certainly would never recognize their children from their descriptions! You may even make a vaguely negative or critical comment about someone's child, possibly even reiterating the mother's own words, only to have her come quickly to the child's defense. You'd better believe I do the same thing when it comes to my "flawless" children.

As a parent I see everything my children are capable of. I know their special abilities and strengths, though these abilities may not shine for everyone they meet. So, in a way, we parents *are* the only qualified experts on our own kids. I have a hard time realizing that my children might not seem so brilliant and gorgeous to everyone else.

✳ ✳ ✳ ✳ ✳

Max asked me again today, "When is Sophie's Down Syndrome going to go away?" Again, I explained it to him as simply as I could.

January 28. When Max and Sophie grow up, Max will probably say, "Mom, I wish you had treated me like a 'special child.' I wish I'd gotten all of that attention." And Sophie will say, "Mom, why didn't you put less attention on my problems and just treat me like a normal child?"

Almost all my gloom has passed. The answer to my question, "Will I ever stop crying?" is *yes!* Somehow I made it through. Some personal counseling helped, along with simply living life—and seeing Sophie grow and become an active, alert baby. She is up on all fours getting ready to crawl—at four and a half months old. This is due to her father's exercise program, the NACD program, and the cross-patterning. Her volunteers come almost every day. Her life is program, program, program. I'm tired of the program, but Sophie shows very good results from it. At some point we have to balance out our lives and the lives of our children, deciding how much time and energy we can spend on each. But for now, our baby's progress is spectacular, and we are tired but thrilled.

January 31. The latest attitude to have is "treat your baby with Down Syndrome like a normal baby." To that I say, "How can we?" First of all, she's in physical therapy twice a week and the NACD program every day. A volunteer comes almost every day to help with cross-patterning. I'm going to begin signing to her as soon as I start class, and she'll be attending speech class one morning a week. Yes, we expect *at least* normal development from her, but we treat her as if her development is an emergency. Yes, we hug and kiss her and laugh with her like any normal baby, but a normal child is not, for the most part, an emergency. Perfectly healthy children have a beautiful, simple, intense, natural drive to accomplish and thrive. In fact they demand it. Sophie's drive is sometimes in low gear or stalled, and we are the ones pushing her uphill by the back bumper. Yes, I have *higher* than normal expectations for her, but I can't treat my child with Down Syndrome completely like a normal child. When I work with Sophie, I sometimes feel like I'm working on a show that's opening in a week with a month's work left to be done.

Today I *do* have dreams for Sophie. I dream of a normal IQ. I dream of standard school placement. I dream of perfect, beautiful speech. I dream of charm and beauty and intelligence. Any parents of a child with disabilities who do not join me in these dreams are doing a disservice to their child, because it's *having the dream itself* that will cause it to come to fruition. That's why it needs to be gently encouraged and nurtured. This is *my* dream and it's valid. The dream itself has value because it changes *me* and in doing so changes my daughter's chances for success. After all, I am her teacher, and she is my responsibility. She'll have the opportunities I expose her to. And I will expose her to those things that I feel she can accomplish or that will challenge her to reach new goals. And I *know* that she will reach every goal we set for her in her own strong and determined way.

February 2. I had a dream two nights ago. I dreamed about a complex of buildings that was a center, a mini-city for children with disabilities. After touring it, I realized it was an old movie studio; the homes and offices had been dressing rooms and bungalows. Plants hung on porches, and a homey and kind feeling pervaded the place. A village rabbi in a blue-gray suit was there to work with the kids and with the parents. He said all perfect things, knew just what everyone was thinking, and generally was a perfect dream of a rabbi or priest or confessor. The environment was one of acceptance and encouragement. Children who came to this village automatically became more articulate and able, because everyone automatically expected it of them. Everyone there had a special ability to understand what the children were saying, and so it seemed they were all doing very well.

You know, it seems that the toughest part of any problem we might run into is going to be dealing with the world, not with Sophie.

February 4. This morning I signed Sophie up for a Mommy and Me class. She wasn't with me. Peter was watching her while I rushed over to be sure we got into the class. It was strange to be in a room full of moms with normal, healthy babies. I realized that my reality has shifted to a point where I'm almost more comfortable in a room filled with problem babies. These children fairly reeked of health. They were perfect, bright-eyed, beautiful little squirts. Again, I longed for Sophie to be healthy.

Later I read an article in *Exceptional Parents* magazine written by the mom of a sixteen-year-old daughter who is mentally retarded. She wrote about how she handled sexuality directly with her child, resulting in more responsible behavior on the part of her daughter. I cried after reading that. My tears came not out of depression, but from a stronger feeling. I realized that we have many challenges ahead and that somehow I need to equip myself and my daughter for them. As Sophie's mother, I am deeply concerned about her future as a young woman. Even as I grow to love her for the sweet, delightful person that she is, it hits me again and again that she is a mystery package. That mystery provides possibilities and hope. Yet at the same time it provides fear and worry. I know I can handle the challenge, but it's a little like jumping into an icy sea with no life preserver.

February 7. Today the results of Sophie's chromosome blood test
came in the mail. I was startled to see an actual copy of a
photograph of her chromosomes. Such a technical, detailed inva-
sion of privacy. I had Sophie's blood drawn for the study when we
went to the City of Hope, so I knew I should expect the results in
about a month. And I knew she had Down Syndrome, so why was
I shocked to see it spelled out so clearly on that innocuous piece of
paper? Trisomy 21. Three chromosomes instead of two on her
twenty-first chromosome section. There was no denying the evidence. I wanted to tear that paper in two and throw it away. I
wanted to make it into a paper airplane and fly it off a hill behind
our house. I wanted to call the lab and tell them they sent the
results to the wrong address, wrong family. Crazily I thought, this
just simply cannot be true. Not my child. There's nothing wrong
with her. Everybody's been fooling me, and now they send me a
counterfeit report to try to convince me that they're right. But
there it was, the inescapable truth on an ugly, sterile document.

February 9. As each day passes, Sophie becomes more "Sophie"
and less "Down Syndrome." Her progress is so great. Today at
almost five months she is scooting slowly but surely across the bed,
the floor, wherever. Her vocalization has picked up, but I still want
more tests done on her hearing. I'm pretty sure her hearing would
be okay were it not affected by the almost constant fluid in her ears.
Right now she's cleared up, and her sounds have increased tenfold.
She's also getting chiropractic adjustments for her ears and for her
sluggish intestines. She seems to be a bit more regular now.
    Her eyes are still blue and her hair's a dark brown, losing some
of its initial auburn tones. Often when Peter is holding and playing
with Sophie I see such a sparkle of love in his eyes; he feels so
strongly about this tot. So often I get such a deep, brief stabbing
feeling of regret, of wishing we were not burdened with all of this.
    Whole days in a row go by with no crying on my part, probably
because I'm too busy to think! My parents were visiting from the
East this week. They were initially so devastated about Sophie.
Now I can tell they see hope and incredible progress and a very cute
baby! Every day she gets better, and so do we. Although I have
emotional setbacks, I'm improving all the time too.

13

She is becoming ours again

We found out that Dr. Turkel's medication, the U-series, is very expensive and is, in fact, unaffordable for us. We are still interested in his theory and have heard of a Canadian pharmacist who has made almost exactly the same medication available for considerably less money. We have asked one of Sophie's many pediatricians for a prescription note for this medication, called the MSB formula, and we are going to send for it. We have researched this thoroughly and have found no reported side effects. Our only concern is that Dr. Turkel will not be monitoring Sophie's progress or her use of the formula. Dr. Turkel says that from what he knows, the MSB formula is not a duplication of his U-series. According to the pharmacist in Canada, it *is* the same, minus any preservatives, fillers, or unnatural colors. So here we are, out on a limb.

Among other things, this medication is supposed to help respiratory problems and chronic congestion. Sophie is so congested today that she can hardly even cough. She has been congestion-free for only about three weeks of her life. When she gets this sick, her progress slows down—we can't take her to Infant Stimulation or do a really thorough NACD program on her. Then she invariably gets an ear infection which affects her hearing, which in turn affects her speech. Dr. H. has said we should get tubes in her ears immediately. We are hoping the MSB formula will work to avoid the need for that operation. These illnesses are not only expensive, they're also very trying because she is so young. She's been on about six courses of antibiotics and has had several ear infections. She must feel uncomfortable a lot of the time, but she always seems so bright and cheerful.

Sophie's ENT doctor says that she is too young for an antihistamine, so how will the cycle ever end?

Frankly, I'm sick of doctors, and so is she!

February 24. We've sent for the MSB formula and are anxiously awaiting its arrival. I hope this helps Sophie.

What a day! I drove Max half an hour each way to preschool. We rushed around in the morning so I could get him there and get to Sophie's Mommy and Me class by 8:30 A.M. There were about twenty-three babies and mothers in the class. We began class by introducing ourselves and telling about the progress of our babies. Sophie is right on schedule with the rest of the babies in her age range. No one in the class indicated in any way that they could tell she had Down Syndrome. Were they just being polite? To me she looks perfect. The moms all voiced mom-like concerns about teething and crawling. I longed to return to the world of "normal" moms with easy questions like that. But I am forever on "the other side," too wise, too old, too watchful and protective of my fragile baby.

The next stop was Jack-in-the-Box, where I picked up junk food on the way to a friend's house. She has a seven-month-old daughter and another friend, who was there too, has a six-week-old baby girl. I felt okay—not sad—around them. I'm becoming more used to Sophie just being a baby, so we were simply moms with babies. The visit was nice. Each of them had saved an article on Down Syndrome for me to read. They were being thoughtful, but for some reason both articles upset me somewhat. The subject is so personal that reading about it in front of other people is hard.

After our visit, I picked up Max at preschool. His neighborhood friend came over to play, and Sophie's cross-patterning volunteer also arrived. We cross-patterned for about half an hour. When she left, Max was still playing so I did most of Sophie's program. I then fed Max, Peter came home, I bathed Max, put Sophie down to sleep, and I got to take a shower! I never thought a shower could feel like a trip to the Bahamas, but this one certainly did.

February 28. I have such mixed feelings about my sign language class. I was sad when I first started the class. Yet as the class goes on, I find I'm really enjoying it. I enjoy a silent language. Now if I can just reconcile myself to why I'm taking it—because Sophie may not speak well—I can give in and enjoy learning. Every sign I learn, I like. It's a very full and exciting language, almost faster than speech and more efficient because a lot of extraneous words are edited. In some ways, it's better than speech because it draws more out of you when you communicate. I use a few basic signs with Sophie like "Mommy," "Papa," "love," "name," and "Sophie," and we sign songs in her Infant Stimulation class. I so clearly remember the feeling of horror and protest when her therapists signed a song to the babies. But I have since learned that speech is the most delayed of all the abilities of these children—not just those children with Down Syndrome, but children with many other kinds of disabilities. In Sophie's speech class, new language lessons are introduced each week. Sometimes these lessons are games and songs to encourage understanding and response—"Patty Cake," "Row, Row, Row Your Boat," "Hokey Pokey." Each week a new word is introduced, like "baby" or "ball." The children are shown the object, told the word for it repeatedly and also taught the sign for the word. Usually a concept, such as "in and out" or "all gone," is also presented. Using signing with delayed children is a relatively new idea, part of what is called "total communication."

At a speech and language class at California State University at Northridge, we heard a lecture on the benefits of teaching a child to sign. A mother spoke of the success she'd had signing with her own Down Syndrome child. The speech-delayed child learns some basic signs to alleviate some of the frustrations that accompany speech problems. As the child begins to speak, he or she no longer uses the signs; they automatically disappear. This makes sense to me. I want to afford Sophie any opportunity to communicate. I can't wait for her first word *or* her first sign!

March 3. Today Sophie and I attended a ladies' luncheon. Of course many of the ladies knew me and knew about Sophie. Each came over to say hello; many were meeting Sophie for the first time. I put Sophie in a pretty dress and she looked adorable. I could see the subtle look of trepidation change to relief and surprise as each new person saw how cute and "normal" she looked. I'm practiced at handling situations like this now. I'm becoming hardened to the fact that we will be educating much of the world we are exposed to, and doing so is less trying each time.

✳ ✳ ✳ ✳ ✳

Sometimes I wonder about the severe cramps and bleeding I
experienced in the twelfth week of my pregnancy with Sophie.
Before Sophie, I'd had a miscarriage; the vehemence of my reaction
over the loss surprised me. I cried bitterly and deeply and felt
bereft for a long time afterward. The miscarriage seemed to take
forever; it was three weeks before the doctor was certain enough to
perform the D and C. I remember sharply the feeling of being
cheated, of hating to visit the obstetrician's office where the walls of
the hallway were lined with pictures of goonie-looking newborns. I
remember the doctor comforting me as I broke down in uncontrollable sobs after the ultrasound showed just a shadow, no fetus.

To me, life in the womb is real, as real as if the baby had already
been born. Ask any pregnant woman whose baby is wanted—is she
carrying life? It is not for me to judge what another woman does,
but for me the termination of pregnancy is the termination of life.

Sometimes I wonder why Sophie lived through that bleeding
episode early in my pregnancy with her. I feel I *willed* her to live
because another miscarriage was unspeakable, unbearable. I feel I
insisted upon her life. I loved her and "knew" it was my daughter
in there. I wanted her; the thought of losing her was not
acceptable. The day after the bleeding I got an ultrasound to check
for signs of life, and there she was: a dancing, kicking peanut! I
was so relieved and felt that a partnership agreement had been
made—you and me, kid, we'll be fine. At the moment of her birth,
I felt a simple certainty confirmed—here's my daughter. She was a
breathtaking gift, ready to unfold. I feel I was brutally robbed of
our gentle evolution together with the necessary influx of doctors,
therapists, programs, lectures, classes, and medications. But I am
slowly reclaiming her. She is becoming ours again.

March 4. The other day one of my close friends told me I "looked
like hell," that I looked "drawn." I was thrilled! All my suffering,
my hard-earned worry lines really show!

You know, you can really milk this deal for all its worth.
Because of my holy dedication to both my son and my "poor little
handicapped baby," I'm getting a lot of applause. I secretly know

that some people are applauding so loudly because they're darn glad they're not in my shoes. I wish I were in the wings with them, watching someone else be noble. I'd love to be clucking over how unbelievable Ms. So-and-So is with her "special" child and how *I*, personally, could *never* handle it.

✳ ✳ ✳ ✳ ✳

Last night my husband and I were reading in bed. Peter had one of his beloved car magazines, and I was attempting to escape into the latest trashy novel. The kids were both sleeping. With his eyes still on the magazine, Peter said, "I love Sophie so much. I wish everything were okay with her." Such a simple statement. Such an absolute, complete truth about our lives for the past six months and for the months and years to come. No matter how much we do for her, all the programs and vitamins in the world can't change the structure of her chromosomes. Ours is such a palpable, mutual helplessness, so intense that we rarely mention it in each other's presence. I can't bear to hear it. I want to make it all better, both for Sophie *and* for her father, who loves her so completely and whose heart is jarred by the slightest setback.

14

Sometimes the pain needs to be shared

March 8. In a few minutes we'll be driving to Children's Hopital to get tubes put in Sophie's ears. She'll need general anesthesia. This worries me. She weighs only about thirteen and a half pounds. Of course yesterday's paper carried a prominent article about a man who went into surgery and was mistakenly injected with some deadly substance. Now he's "brain dead." Why is it that moms always see these articles?

I know Sophie needs these tubes. Taking so many antibiotics for her chronic ear infections has got to be taking it's toll on her already sluggish immune system.

9:05 A.M. I'm sitting in the lobby of Children's Hospital waiting for Sochie to be called in for surgery. Most of the children in this waiting area are visibly impaired or sick or are here for surgery. One little boy in a wheelchair has cerebral palsy. Another boy has scars on his head from previous surgery. Some just have kid things—bandages on hands, tonsil problems, or whatever. Although no one is talking, I feel an undercurrent of tension and anxiety, shared by all of the parents. But we are all pretending that everything is as it should be. Are we pretending for our children or for our own benefit?

9:45 A.M. The mystery of what exactly will occur in the operating room keeps me from trusting the doctor, the procedure, and the whole place. Allowing my child to be wheeled away on a gurney makes me feel like a fool. What if something goes wrong? I've reassured myself a hundred times that everything's going to be fine. Well, so far no gurney. We're still waiting to talk with the anesthesiologist.

10:15 A.M. A nurse took Sophie. We were able to accompany her
only as far as the elevator. Leaving her there, instead of walking
with her to the operating room, was horrible. There's probably no
sensitive way to take away someone's baby for an operation.
Sophie's surgery is such a small procedure; I know I'm overreact-
ing. Because she will be anesthetized, I feel that I have given
someone else the power of life or death over my baby.

Dr. Jeffery Birns, Sophie's ENT who will put in the ear tubes,
spent time with me in his office prior to the surgery and answered
all my questions without condescension. He gave Sophie a very
thorough examination. I felt he was competent as well as concerned. He treated both Sophie and me like real people. I just
wish I could see him now, for reassurance.

We have asked three times to see the anesthesiologist, once before
our hospital visit. A few minutes ago I was able to talk with him
over the hospital phone, but I'm surprised that I couldn't see him
face to face. He told me what the procedure would involve: gas, a
muscle relaxant, and a tube in her trachea. No big deal to him, but
to us it's quite a tall order for a six-month-old infant. He sounded
a bit impatient. It frustrates me to be so dependent upon these
professionals, whom 99 percent of the population seem to treat as if
they walk on water.

12:50 P.M. Sophie is out of the operating room! I got to hold her in
the recovery room and nurse her. What a relief to see her! She
was sweet and sleepy. She lived through it, and so did we! Dr.
Birns came to see me in the recovery room and suddenly all my
tension lifted. He had saved my baby from the brink of death! He
may have only put tubes in her ears, but it felt like major surgery to
me! The operation went well, he told me. There was a lot of fluid
in her ears that could not have been detected with office instruments
and never would have drained properly without the surgery. He
reassured us that the surgery had been beneficial; he added that her
hearing should improve and infections should clear up immediately.

We are both relieved and pleased. So now, of course, *we* are
numbered among that ninety-nine percent who think all doctors
walk on water!

On the way home from the hospital we stopped at the post office to pick up the MSB formula from Canada (the Canadian pharmacist's version of the U-series). We're confused because the formula differs in ingredients and in some of the amounts from the original U-series created by Dr. Turkel. I need to call the Canadian company that makes it and find out why.

We have an appointment on March 22 with the famous Professor Schmid to discuss cell therapy. I'm at the point where I want to get Sofe going on all these treatments so I don't have to think about them anymore!

At least now I don't have to think about tubes! Sophie finally has them. Dr. H. will be thrilled, since she's the one who pushed for them. I have a hunch that Sophie's vocalization will improve as she's able to hear a little better.

We continue every day with her NACD program. She is crawling a lot on her tummy, even across the room. She's also more stable on all fours and rocks back and forth when she gets up there. This position is called "four point" in her physical therapy program, but I call it her "get-up-and-go" position. She really looks cute and babylike when she's like that.

Her papa calls her Sweetie Bear. And that's what she is.

March 10. Today Max and I went to a Purim carnival at the Temple while Peter stayed with Sochie at home. This is the third or fourth event we've attended at the Temple since Sophie's birth. These visits seem to be the last bastion of that swallow-back-my-tears feeling. The Temple activities, more than any other, sadden me. The inequity of our situation hits me harder there, where I see so many cute little girls. Moms bring their infant or toddler daughters to the Temple carnival. Daughters in new dresses dance to the holiday songs. Families show off their children.

I'm just beginning to know some of these people, and I really like a lot of them. But my life has a little twist beyond the normal craziness that everyone experiences.

Even though mine was not a religious upbringing, we followed some traditions and always had a close family feeling. It's important and exciting to me to pass those traditions on to my children. But can I do this with Sophie?

March 12. When I first started this diary, it was a place to pour out all my terrible feelings. As curious as many people are, I knew that no one really wanted to hear as much as I wanted to say. No one asked. No one really knew I had these feelings, I guess. Some things feel better left unshared, as if sharing them will give strength to the reality you're trying to dispel instead of lightening the load. Then, as time passed, a couple of people said to me, "You should write down some of your experiences." And I thought, I already am, but does anybody really want to *read* them?

At some point I decided maybe other parents in my shoes would read this. I hope so, because sometimes the pain needs to be shared.

Sometimes I picture what other parents in our situation might be going through. Peter and I have a strong marriage. Each of us is the other's best friend and, all in all, we have the wherewithal to survive this crisis. What do other couples do? How can they be handling this? Those we know seem to present a relaxed facade, so who knows what they really feel?

Oh—some good news. Max was talking about Dinky today, so I asked a few more questions about him. "Where is Dinky?" "What can Dinky do?" Max answered me impatiently in his "important" voice, "Mommy, don't you even know that Dinky is *imaginary*? That means he's not really here. I made him up!"

Whew.

15

We're learning to travel our own path

March 14. We are thinking of taking Sophie out of Infant Stimulation. I know the physical therapy is necessary for her development, to some degree. I also understand that it has to be body-oriented. But my child is more than a body, and I can't stand to treat her like a roly-poly doll. Even though the therapy may be beneficial, I feel that treating Sophie this way, in this kind of environment, may outweigh the benefits. Too much emphasis is placed on the disability. Being around so many disabled babies is hard for me and feels wrong for Sophie.

I have always been uncomfortable about the therapy in Infant Stimulation, yet I fear dropping out of the acceptable process of handling my child. It's scary to wonder if we're giving up something impulsively and will learn later we should have kept on with it. Will we also be giving up contacts with the other mothers or the support group? Or risking disapproval within the medical and therapeutic community of which my child has become an inextricable part? I just can picture the case report: "Mother chose to withdraw child from Infant Stimulation against advice of physical therapist. We feel at this time the mother is being unrealistic about the child's future and about her ability to handle the child on her own."

Who are these people, anyway, who seem to have power over my child and my family?

March 16. We're definitely taking "the Sofe" out of Infant Stimulation. I've written notes to the therapists, and I feel great about it. It's a reclamation! We can raise our own child and do fine. We'll continue with the NACD program, the MSB formula, and Dr. H.'s B_6. We're learning to travel our own path—a rocky one—but we're getting better and better at it. Peter and I talked a lot about this decision and feel it is totally right for all of us.

Over the last month Sophie has lost one and a half pounds. This weight loss began before the MSB formula, so we've ruled that out as a cause. We think it may be the fact that she's eating the same amount but scooting all over like a wild woman. She's showing a little interest in solid foods now. What a relief! At six months, she's still only nursing! She *loves* to nurse. That's fine, except at 3:00 in the morning—not my favorite time to be awake.

Next week we meet with Professor Schmid about cell therapy. I've already found a certified professional to administer the cells, should we decide to go for it.

✵ ✵ ✵ ✵ ✵

I'm learning so much. I think there are alternatives to some special education settings, especially for kids with Down Syndrome— depending on each child's capabilities, of course. It may be time for a revolution or a civil war between parents and professionals. How can a professional learn about my child from a book? Or from college? Or from teachers? They can only learn about my child two ways—from her parents and from Sophie. There are no better sources. Tell that to most doctors, therapists, or professors, and you've got a silent—sometimes not so silent—war on your hands. Some of the professional attitudes I've encountered would make your hair stand on end. I know that my search for competent and gentle and *interested* professionals for my child's care will probably never end. But I also can see that one of my goals is going to be to eliminate all but the most necessary and most able of these people from our lives. This will be a trick, because often we are dependent upon them for things we cannot do ourselves.

March 20. Well, on the first day of spring I'm sitting alone outside in my backyard. The sun is bright and warm. The sky is exactly as it should be in California, blue and clear, calling half the popula- tion of the state to the beach. Sophie is napping and Max is playing fairly quietly, occasionally pestering me for a drink or a snack. Sophie woke up only twice last night instead of the usual four or five times, so I feel relatively rested.

This morning the question of whether or not to have another baby popped into my mind. I wanted to be finished after Sophie. During my endless, uncomfortable pregnancy with her, I spoke to Peter several times about the possibility of a vasectomy. At the time I was irritated by what I thought was his silly response, "No one's doing anything to cut *me* up!" But now I'm glad he was so stubborn.

Because of our unexpected circumstances with Sophie, I'm pretty certain I want a third child. The reasons float through my head, my thoughts fighting with one another: Maybe Sophie won't be all a sibling should be for Max. Then the answer: Too bad! Sophie *is* Max's sibling and I know that he will love her just as much as he would love any sister. Will it be too great a burden on Max to be his sister's eventual caretaker, without having any other siblings to pitch in? Same answer: Too bad! Life places certain burdens on all of us, and it's our responsibility to take them on, whether or not they are easy. I hope we can instill this value in Max. There's no guarantee that a third sibling would agree to carry out those responsibilities. There's not even a guarantee that Max will.

Another thought immediately enters my head. Our initial plan was to have two able-bodied, able-minded children, and we didn't reach that goal. Then I answer myself: Too bad! Sophie is our whole, beautiful daughter, just as she is. And having a third child isn't going to change her, anyway. My discourse with myself continues: If I get pregnant again so soon, people will think we don't love our daughter and are trying to replace her with another baby. Then comes my immediate answer: Too bad! We *do* love her.

Other thoughts rumble around: I dread the very exhausting time of the first few months after the birth, when the baby is not sleeping and is completely dependent upon me for food. I follow with: Too bad! The hard times are finite and my biological clock is running out. It's now or never.

I may have talked myself into it. Now let's see if Peter will come to the same conclusion.

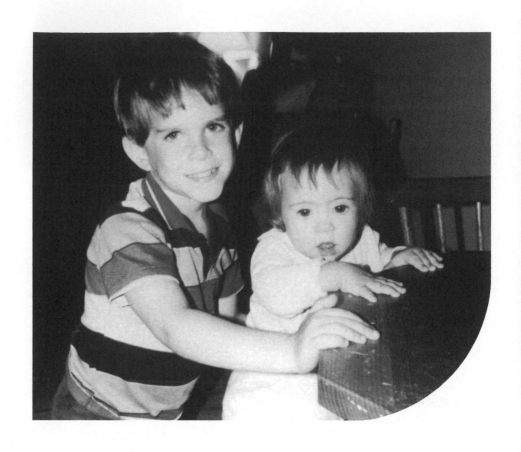

16

I thought Sophie could never be
beautiful, but she is!

March 23. Several months ago, when we went to the seminar on
alternative methods of treatment for symptoms of Down Syndrome,
we learned about cell therapy. Since then we have been doing
research on the subject through a group of people who support the
therapy. Through their newsletter, we heard that Dr. Schmid is
going to be in the United States soon and that, in exchange for a
contribution to his airfare, we could have an appointment with him
while he was here. We were intrigued and very interested in
consulting with this man about our daughter. We also knew that
this arrangement would save us a trip to Germany. We were
interested in possibly trying one injection for Sophie, and we
wanted to meet the famous doctor about whom we had heard and
read so much. We decided to send in the donation and get our
appointment with him.

So, after waiting many weeks, we met with Dr. Schmid yesterday.
We had been sent directions to his temporary office in a hotel and
were instructed not to reveal the location, for fear that other parents
without appointments would try to see this busy physician. The
hotel was about one and a half hours from our home. After the
long drive with the kids, we finally arrived and were told by the desk
clerk to wait in the lobby. After about fifteen minutes, a woman
came up to us and explained that Dr. Schmid was running a little
behind schedule. Three or four other sets of parents of children
with Down Syndrome were also waiting in the lobby. We were all
very quiet, sensing that this was somehow confidential.

Our wait was an anxious one, because we had no idea whether or
not Sophie would actually be receiving a cell injection that day

during the appointment. The illegal aspect of the cell therapy in the
United States cloaked the meeting in mystery.

Finally a second woman called our name and led us through the
halls to Dr. Schmid's small temporary office. Peter and I both were
slightly uncomfortable with the hush-hush nature of the entire
episode, but we had come this far and wanted to meet the doctor.
When we entered his tiny office, we encountered a kindly, white-
haired Santa Claus *sans* beard. He spoke briefly with Max, teasing
him a little in a nice way, and then fell silent, almost as if he'd
forgotten we were there. I cleared my throat and asked him some
questions about the therapy itself, some of its risks and procedures.
He answered very intelligently in a thickly accented voice. He
reviewed the written medical history that we had filled out beforehand and asked us questions to clarify some aspects of what we had
written down. Unless we initiated the conversation, though, he had
almost nothing to say. Both Peter and I felt so strange, as if we
were uninvited guests. He sat there writing notes on Sophie's
medical history. He asked us if we were familiar with cell therapy.
After we assured him that we were, he explained to us how to
obtain the cells in Germany. No mention was made of how they
were to be injected. The doctor was obviously very well informed
on his subject and thoroughly competent in deciding who would
benefit from it. He told us that he himself took the injections for
their rejuvenating qualities, and he did indeed look younger than his
years and very healthy.

The appointment lasted for a total of about twenty minutes.
After leaving the hotel we discussed our strange feelings. Although
we could not pinpoint the reason, the whole day was disquieting.

Despite our respect for Dr. Schmid's work in the area of
improving the physical and mental development of many children
with Down Syndrome, we still felt degraded after meeting with him.
We knew this feeling was not necessarily a reflection on the doctor's
success in his field. It's likely that when he is in his own country,
where his treatment is not only legal but highly respected, this
"underground" feeling doesn't exist. Actually, nothing illegal had
happened; this was simply a consultation. No mention was made
of Sophie receiving the injection that day. Still, we were uncom-

fortable enough with the encounter to give ourselves more time before making our final decision about a cell injection.

March 24. Every time I see a child in public who has Down Syndrome, I want to run up to the mother and say, "Oh! My baby has Down Syndrome too!" I find that, because we love Sophie so much, we consider everything about her beautiful and outstanding. So when I see a child who is in some way like Sophie, I'm delighted! I'm beginning to think babies with Down Syndrome are especially pretty because my baby is so cute! It's a new viewpoint and a positive one, even if it is a little weird.

March 25. Tonight I feel sad, and I'm not sure why. I am exhausted and feel that all my efforts are useless and that they rob me of my vitality and happiness. At some point in the future I may expand Sophie's volunteer program so that the volunteers can do her entire NACD program with her. I don't want to be Therapy Mommy, I want to be Peek-a-Boo Mommy and Hugs-and-Kisses Mommy. What I'd really like is for all this worry and therapy to go away.

Fantasy: Sophie comes running into the room when she's sixteen years old and says, "Mom, I was just thinking about the time I had Down Syndrome. Wasn't that a heck of a trial for all of us? Just think—if they hadn't found a cure, I'd still have it."

But the truth is that there *is* no cure. This is forever. Her fate is sealed. I can't seem to shake the feeling that her blueprint has been set, and much of our running around is pure puppetry for our own satisfaction and distraction.

Sometimes I know I'm too tired and disheartened to have a third child. Then I stop and think that any mother with two young kids might feel that way!

March 27. Today was Sophie's first re-evaluation with NACD. What an exciting and happy event. We were so proud of our scooting baby. Everyone wanted to hold her. It's really a great place, and it feels good to be connected with the people there.

Bob Doman revised her program. No more ramp! Sophie has graduated! We still need to do the cross-patterning until her

crawling pattern is "cross" and not "homologous." We're supposed to expose her to two or three hours of music and songs and
taped vowel sounds every day. We're going to start work on her
"cortical opposition" (otherwise known as picking up little stuff
with her thumb and first finger), and there are other changes too.
We're told to have her crawl over two-by-four boards about one and
a half inches high, do some spinning with her, expose her to more
tastes and odors, keep showing and naming objects around the
house (this we do naturally anyway), mimic her sounds, continue to
show her picture cards, and try to cover her mouth so that she gets
used to breathing through her nose. This last part is a little tough
since, first of all, she hates it and, second of all, her nose is often
stuffed so we can't do it!

Max came with us and, although a little restless, he behaved
fairly well. I'm not sure if it's wise to take him along to sessions
like this one, where Sophie gets all the attention, or if it's better to
leave him at a friend's house, where he might feel excluded from
our outings with Sophie. Who knows? We're pioneering—and so
is he!

When Sophie was first born, I had so many confused thoughts. I
thought all people with Down Syndrome looked alike, regardless of
their families. I thought Sophie had different "genes" and
wouldn't look like us. But she does look like us, just like every
other little girl looks like her parents. I thought Sophie could never
be beautiful. But she *is* beautiful, not just to me, but to lots of
people I don't even know who compliment her in public.

I thought her eyes were different because of the "Brushfield
spots" associated with Down Syndrome. But her eyes are denim
blue and wide and round and expressive and *hers*, regardless of her
darned chromosomal pattern.

I read that her hair would be thin, stringy, and brown. Her hair
is soft, full, and chestnut. I love to wash it and brush it with her
baby brush.

I thought maybe she'd always be sleepy and slow and unresponsive. She is alert, knows me and her papa very well, loves and
adores her brother, and responds to friends but is hesitant to smile
at strangers, which shows excellent discrimination. We are learning

from Sophie that not everything written in books or told to us by doctors is true. She is helping us break through our own ignorance.

March 30. Peter's paternal family background has been a bit of a mystery because he hasn't seen his natural father since age twelve. His mother says she knows little of his father's past life and was never closely acquainted with his relatives. She remarried a wonderful man when Peter was very young, and Peter's stepfather, John, really brought him up. When I was pregnant with Max, I suddenly wanted Peter's birth father to know us and for us to know him. We knew only the name of the town and state where he grew up. With the aid of Directory Assistance, we found people with Peter's original last name and we wrote to them. It turns out they *were* related to him and were delighted we had contacted them. There were aunts, uncles, and many cousins—all happily ensconced in the Midwest. None of them, however, knew where Peter's father was and were just as baffled as we were by his disappearance from his entire family so many years ago.

There began a correspondence between us and these relatives. Photographs were exchanged, family histories and relationships explained. Yesterday we received a letter from Peter's cousin's family. We hadn't told them right away about Sophie's problems, just about her birth. They sent congratulations and a delicate gold heart necklace. About a month later I sent out the newsletter that described the situation. It must have touched a deep and responsive chord in our "new" cousin, because she wrote of a child she had given birth to and whom she had lost. The girl was only fourteen days old when she died, a result of complications from multiple congenital physical problems. I guess some things are kept secret not because you are hiding them but because they are too difficult and personal to share. But I'm glad Peter's cousin shared this with us. A real bond is created between mothers when something goes wrong with the births or lives of their children.

April 2. I have been thinking about why I acted the way I did when Sophie was born. I shared my real feelings with no one except my husband. Except for one or two times when I couldn't stop myself, I cried only when I was alone.

My constant unhappiness was so intensely personal, I did not want to share it. I felt it was wrong to be unhappy about my own baby.

Those times I did cry in front of others, I didn't feel relieved. I just felt mortified. I'm not at ease with weepy people, and I somehow felt that people would back off if I fell apart publicly.

Also, I knew deep down that there wasn't a thing they could do, so why put them in an even more helpless position?

I was so miserable most of the time that I preferred to be alone so that I didn't have to be sociable and coherent.

Though the sadness is still there, I'm glad that I no longer feel such overwhelming grief, that I've returned to a semblance of sanity.

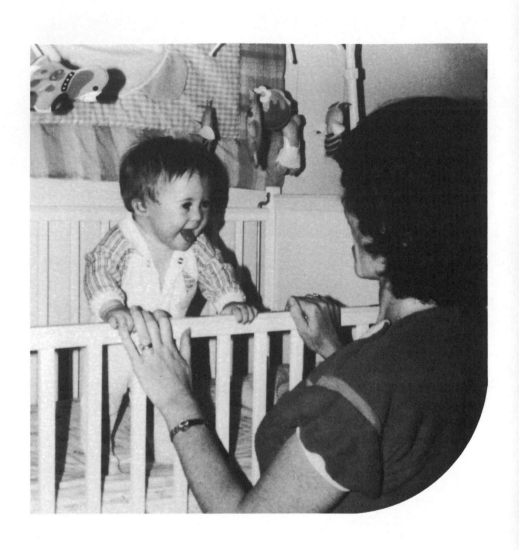

17

Slowly, slowly, my days are getting brighter

April 6. We're at my aunt's cabin at Arrowhead, where it's quiet and peaceful. This is really our first family vacation since Sophie's birth. The lack of everyday distractions is both relaxing and disquieting. For some reason life is easier for me to handle when it's filled with distractions. Distractions from what? From melancholy, from the truth, from my subtle sorrow. With such quiet around me, the sadness sneaks back.

Last week I took Sophie back to the Infant Stimulation program for their annual "Alumni Day." Activities were planned for children of all ages who were coming back to visit their "school." At the end of the day's activities, current and past students were all assembled into a circle for song time. As I observed these children with my pasted-on smile, I noticed how overly jolly I must seem—a social reaction to my real shock and pain at seeing so many disabled children. Some were more severely disabled than others. Again, Down Syndrome seemed to be a gift when I saw those tiny kids in specially designed wheelchair-strollers, or one child who was just lying down, totally noncommunicative and very tiny for her five years.

Afterward, as I was driving out of the parking lot, I realized again that, although the therapy may be excellent, it's not necessary to put all the kids with problems in one place like some unnecessary club. It's true that some of the children are so impaired that placing them in other situations is not easy. It's also true that the kids and families who have been involved in this program know one another and enjoy the reunion. I understand that. We are lucky that Sophie is doing as well as she is. But because she's doing well,

I believe that Mommy and Me classes, our home program, and many other normal activities would benefit her just as much. We don't need to immerse ourselves in "the disability" any more than is absolutely necessary; it's overwhelming as it is.

April 8.   I go through stages of up and down. Yesterday a friend of mine from college days called. I was surprised and delighted to hear from her. She asked about Sophie, saying, "I'm sorry about your little girl. Is she with you at home?" I was so taken aback by the question I just answered, "Oh, yes!" What I wanted to say was, "How could you ask me that? What are you talking about?"

Later in the conversation she asked, "Are you very confined with her?" implying that she thought Sophie probably had a much more severe disability that she actually has. I hadn't realized the extent of the public's lack of awareness about Down Syndrome. My day was ruined by her question, "Is she with you at home?" A question like that breaks my heart in two, no matter how gently it is asked. Later, when I told my mother about this question, she confessed that others had asked her similar questions about Sophie. "Are they going to keep her?" "Is she at home?" My mother's answer to them was "Well, it's a little soon to send her out to work!"

About two days ago, while I was giving Sophie her program, a thought about her came to me, sudden and unbidden: "How could you do this to me?" I felt it so strongly, and at the same time I was shocked that I could have that thought about my own baby. I felt so resentful and sorry that she had Down Syndrome, that our future as mother and daughter was so up in the air. I *don't want* a retarded daughter. Yet now, as I look at her, I don't see a retarded daughter, but a beautiful, active, bright-eyed little pickle! She is normal in her development; so far, she is fine. Still, I can't seem to chase away fears of the future and regrets over the loss of my "normal" daughter. Sometimes I get listless and unable to love Sophie completely.

Soon she will be seven months old. With each passing month my fears grow—fear that her retardation will show now that she's supposed to be doing this or that, fear that her features might become unattractive, fear that as she approaches one year of age, the world and my family will begin to see what we have been subtly denying: seriously delayed development.

I don't think any parent can believe it until it's happening before their eyes. And even then it's not obvious to them because this is simply the way their child is. When a delay does become apparent, it is never as shocking as the imaginary fears you have had about it beforehand, because this is your child whom you've always known and loved. This slow evolution can almost make such disabilities invisible to a parent.

April 14. Sophie's speech has improved one hundred percent. It's so neat to hear her authentic baby sounds!

April 17. Yesterday was a quiet day—no classes or doctors for either Max or Sophie! We stayed home, working on Sophie's program, playing, cleaning the house. It was nice—a regular mom-and-kids day. My friend Raye and her two-month-old daughter came over to visit. We were both pregnant at the same time with our girls. She has two sons and had been dreaming of a daughter. Her daughter is so alive, so vital and healthy—without any program! My daughter is vital and energetic and progressing "on target" too, but of course it hasn't been the same process. Where her daughter has brought her nothing but joy and sparkling love, my daughter's arrival brought me the greatest pain I have ever known. I cannot honestly say that all the pain has subsided and has been replaced with unbounded joy. No, I can't say that.

But slowly, slowly, my days are getting brighter.

April 19. On Thursday a new friend and I took our children to McDonald's for a gourmet feast of burgers, Chicken McNuggets, and fries. I had an opportunity to talk with her six-year-old son, David, who has Down Syndrome, and observe him while he ate and played with the other kids. My spirit was lifted for the rest of the day! This little guy was not only cute but bright, talkative, and as physically coordinated as any kid his age. And, of course, he was in love with McDonald's hamburgers. He was well mannered, sociable, a little devilish, confident, and active. He and Max played together on all the equipment in the playground—the slide, merry-go-round, and bouncing fish. Watching David helped wipe away a lot of grim thoughts.

David's mother, Suzanne, has placed him in a normal school environment, not in a special education setting. She worked with cross-patterning him when he was younger too. She also works with him for two hours each day on academics. For whatever reason, David is thriving.

As the days pass I'm feeling more strongly opposed to the special education environment. I don't feel it will be appropriate or helpful to Sophie. The NACD concept includes the statement that it is better to keep your child home than to place him or her in a special education class. Everything I observe reinforces this concept. This approach is not for every mother of every student, I know. But so far it is for me, and Peter agrees wholeheartedly. Keeping Sophie out of special education and providing her with the finest education possible will be an interesting challenge. But that kind of thing is my forte. And I'm not alone. I'm meeting a network of parents who are keeping their kids either at home or in regular school programs. These kids seem to be doing the best of all those whom I've observed.

✳ ✳ ✳ ✳ ✳

I'm finding out that the term "mainstreaming" means different things to different people. To many uninitiated parents of children with disabilities, it means sending their children to regular school with nondisabled kids. It means their child is actually *in classes* with normal children, exposed to all the ups and downs of a standard, hectic, varied, exciting, and challenging education.

My friend JoAnn recently attended a seminar on special education offered at UCLA by teachers, lawyers, parent and child advocates, and special education administrators. JoAnn has an eleven-month-old baby with Down Syndrome, and we are pioneering together through the vast and mysterious network of activities available to our children. She told me that *she* learned mainstreaming meant, according to the school district, that all the special-needs kids are rounded up in special education classes on a public school campus. They share recess time and cafeteria space with other students. There is some advocacy done about these special-needs kids with the nondisabled kids in such situations as school assemblies. The special kids are given instructions and lessons according to their IEP (Individualized Educational Program). Each school and class is different, of course. Depending upon whom you're talking to, these classes are either "fantastic, helpful and educational" or "glorified baby sitting." I guess I have a lot to learn.

Obviously no one is completely happy about having an impaired child. Any parent is bound to be angry and sad and resentful about the fact that his or her child may need extra help in school. But this does not mean that a parent is also powerless and must agree to letting a possibly educable child be herded into a trainable mentally retarded class simply because that's the school district's policy, or because a psychologist has recommended it. To segregate such children from others can lead to isolation and further developmental delays.

I know it is difficult to give more attention to one child than to the others in a classroom. I, for one, am willing to develop a volunteer program of teacher's aides to work with my daughter if need be. Maybe I can actually have some control over her education, who knows?

But I think I'm getting ahead of myself here.

I'll probably change my mind two hundred times about this whole subject before Sophie is of school age.

April 24. At seven and one half months, Sophie is finally on solid food. She is, however, still nursing up a storm and gaining lots of weight.

Yesterday she pulled herself to standing on my knee! Also, her crawl was a tiny bit in a cross-pattern. I held my breath when I saw that. Four months of daily cross-patterning with volunteers is paying off! Today she did the same things again! She's also been sleeping through the night for the past week. Hurray!

My son has a reddish eyeball, which the doctor said was an infection. So every four hours Max and I battle it out with eye drops.

Today I guiltily but happily bought four or five paperback books spontaneously off the rack in a bookstore. I eagerly read the bulk of one and got the gist of another.

Books are a great, acceptable, legal, even lauded way of total escape. They are my only addiction (besides chocolate chip danishes, pound cake, and extra-rich ice cream). I like to *own* my books, feel them, bend down the corners to keep my place (a cardinal sin according to my mother), write phone numbers on the insides of the covers. And, when I'm finished reading them, I like to give them away to someone with whom I want to share that particular adventure or experience (provided I no longer need the phone numbers). Books are like secret friends who share themselves totally and never argue with you. Why isn't the rest of life like that?

April 27. Today Max had a piano lesson. Afterward we got sandwiches from a Greek deli and brought them home to eat. All of us puttered around the house. I helped Max learn to ride his Hot Wheels, and Peter built some climbing boards for Sophie's program.

My aunt called to tell us that my cousin's baby was born! A girl, Amanda. I was very happy for her and for my cousins. They already have a boy and, although they never said anything, I think they really wanted a girl. My aunt said to me, "Now we all have granddaughters and daughters and can all go out together on Mother's Day for our special luncheon!" My dream exactly. I congratulated her. As I hung up the phone I was ashamed of my real reaction. I felt empty, depressed, deprived. I surprised myself; I guess I didn't know I'd react this way. I knew my cousin was pregnant and that her baby was due any minute. I had feelings only of excitement and anticipation until I heard the baby was born—until I heard it was a girl. I feel so excluded from that club of celebrating, happy, new mothers. And I feel so small for feeling that way. My victories seem slight compared to the victory of giving birth to a healthy child.

I wish I had nothing to write about in this journal. I wish my life were too uncomplicated to be of interest, too ordinary, too simple.

April 29. Right now Max is napping, and Sophie is playing with the bells in her crib. So often I feel I am putting in tremendous effort for Sophie and still she progresses very slowly. True, she is "combat crawling," her vocalization has improved, she stands when you hold her hands, she crawls over obstacles that are four or five inches high, she can keep herself in a standing position while holding on to the coffee table with both hands. For some reason it is getting harder for me—not easier—to do all this work and then see healthy babies her age. They are getting older and progressing by leaps and bounds, while Sophie seems so delicate, fragile, and slower than they are. I should be thinking about other things but my mind seems to be invaded with a buzzing army of thoughts about Down Syndrome.

Today I read that many adults with Down Syndrome after the age of thirty-five develop Alzheimer's Disease. So again I am reminded that Down Syndrome can be a progressive problem. With Sophie, we're on the up side now. As tediously difficult as her program is, she is at least *improving*, getting smarter, becoming more able. Who knows what the future holds? Will Sophie eventually stop getting better, or is that a myth too?

My whole purpose as a parent is to help my kids improve and thrive. So far, so good. I've been relentlessly sad over the past month or so, maybe because I see that this problem is not going away, no matter *how* hard we work!

May 2. Right now Peter, Max, Sophie, and I are all in our bed together. Peter is singing to Sophie. Max is lying next to me on my pillow. Very sweet. I love this bunch of humans who are gathered around me.

18

I now have a baby,
not a project

May 4. We've stopped giving Sophie her program—stopped the
volunteers and the cross-patterning. I had been telling Peter how
depressed I was, that Sophie was not benefiting visibly in proportion
to the amount of work she and I were doing, for the five months I
have spent administering Sophie's program and working with her
volunteers. So Peter and I talked and talked and talked some
more.

We felt the program had been effective in her development up to
this point, yet we realized that our baby also needs fresh air, some
time to be a baby, some time to accomplish on her own. We have
been so frightened by her past lethargy, her seeming inability to
develop at her own pace that we hadn't noticed that the fire had
already been lit; she is developing beautifully. We have a constant
fear of regression or perhaps of "allowing" her to slow down in her
development. But you know what? I know my baby. She is
thriving now and will continue to thrive on her own. For the past
four days we've stopped the program altogether. What a relief!
Not only is my baby doing well, but so am I! Instead of the
program, we take walks, read books, visit friends, lie out in the
sun. Sophie and I are working on our tans. (We have the same
coloring.) I can almost sense the relief in her. If she could speak, I
know she would be saying, "Thanks for letting me be, Mom!" I
now have a baby, not a project. I don't feel tired or sad. I feel
happy. We are all doing better.

May 7. Last night Peter and I attended a meeting at Sophie's
Speech and Language class. Peter saw a videotape of Sophie in

class, and now he's enthused about coming to a class. That would be fun!

This was the third day I've been able to give Sophie her MSB formula. She now eats enough solid food so that I can slip the formula into her food and disguise the taste. After breakfast and her morning dose of this mixture (she gets two doses each day), she began to move around and yell and smile with so much energy I was worried that some amphetamines had accidentally been mixed with the vitamins! Some of the ingredients of the formula have stimulant properties but all are natural and harmless—not like caffeine or another type of direct stimulant, as explained to me by the chemist who made it up. He reassured me that the formula contained every ingredient that was in the U-series except for the fillers, colors, a few modifications in vitamin dosages, and one updated version of an older drug that was in the U-series.

According to the creator of the U-series, Dr. Turkel, this medication is supposed to alleviate some symptoms of Down Syndrome—physical as well as mental. I'm going to try to be as objective as possible in my observations, but objectivity is difficult for two reasons: everything Sophie does seems great to us because she's our baby, and also I'm so eager for positive results that I'll probably be looking extra hard for little changes.

So much for the scientific approach.

May 12. Mother's Day. I joined my cousins, sister, and aunt for an elegant brunch. We had a great time. Peter watched Sophie and my cousin's husband watched Max. Sophie can go without nursing for several hours now. What a relief that is! She doesn't drink well from a cup yet, so I'm still her only real source of anything to drink. It was nice to be free and relaxed and enjoying myself in an adult environment. I only felt a few stabs of sadness as I saw young, prettily-dressed, bright, sassy daughters joining their moms for this special day. I know Sophie will join us too someday.

Tonight Max was playing a make-believe game by himself, complete with explosion sounds and violent language: "I got you! You're dead!" The standard war play every mother knows *her* child would *never* indulge in. At some point during this mighty battle he turned to me and said, "Only mean guys die, right, Mommy?"

"Right," I said, cheating him of a more truthful answer because I wanted to get back to my magazine. Only mean guys die, I thought to myself. And bad things only happen to mean, awful people. And apples come from Johnny Appleseed. And if only Donna Reed married Father Knows Best all would be well.

May 20. I'm in the process of weaning Sophie and today was her first day of no nursing. She survived nicely. It was hard not to give in to her when she nuzzled her tiny cheeks against me, but I was strong!

I have to wean her before I get pregnant again, which we have planned for July. You heard right. Pregnant. Our final reasons? Because we want a third child, regardless. And because it's now or never. Tomorrow I will be thirty-three. And also because we want a majority of healthy kids to balance out all of our lives.

It's funny how, as each day goes by, Sophie is more and more my perfect baby and less and less Down Syndrome. That is, if depression doesn't grip me and talk me out of it.

May 22. For my birthday my sweet husband, whom I love above all others in the universe, took me to dinner and a movie and bought me a book. We were away from the kids for *five hours*! I really felt like a grown-up. Weaning a baby is as much a thrill as it is a heartbreak. Independence is the thrill. And independence is the heartbreak.

May 23. I went to the dentist today because a big chunk fell out of a molar. Sophie came with me in her stroller and was a good, sweet baby the whole time. Sometime during the laborious process of preparing my molar for a crown the dentist asked me, "Has she been a good baby?"

Although I usually avoid the subject with people who don't need to know, for some reason I said, "Well, she was born with Down Syndrome so she has been a hard baby."

He said, "Gee, she doesn't look Down's." And then he casually added, "I have a son with Down's."

"Really?" I exclaimed, delighted to find a heretofore undiscovered ally. "How old is he?"

"Ten," the dentist answered.

When I asked if his son was in school, he said, "Yes, you know, in the special program in the public schools. He's very delayed." He didn't offer any further information.

A little later, after he removed some green Martian goo he had clamped in the far reaches of my mouth, I asked, "Did he have heart problems?"

"No. He had those seizures. We got him one of those . . . uh . . . EEGs and found out he has one every five minutes. He's kind of in a daze."

I was digesting this information while biting down on a strip of pink wax when he added, "He's with a foster parent now. She only has Down's kids. Right now she has three other Down's kids."

"Oh," I said.

And then all of a sudden he was in a hurry and had the dental assistant finish up.

This whole discussion blasted me out of my very recent thoughts about the probable onset of a full set of dentures.

Before Sophie came, I would have automatically judged this man to be horrible, but now I've learned that sometimes things are not as absolute as I'd like to think. I couldn't tell whether his offhand manner was because he really wasn't emotionally involved or whether it was such a source of upset in his life that he'd adopted a casual facade. Although I don't know all of the facts and it's none of my business, the niggling thought remains: how could this family have sent their child to foster care?

✳ ✳ ✳ ✳ ✳

My friend Michelle, a devout Catholic for all of her twenty-four years, suddenly stopped reading her Bible after her first child, a son, was born with Down Syndrome. She told me she was very angry and that many of her firmly held beliefs had been shattered. Not only had she lost her dream of a healthy son, she had lost the foundation of her life: her religion and her unwavering belief that God would be good to those who served Him well.

Most parents suddenly revert to a somewhat different version of the "foxhole theory" when confronted with the unanswerable question, "Why my child?" Instead of fervent prayer suddenly springing from our lips, there occurs instead fervent anger at a God that some of us were not even sure existed.

In our life adventure with Sophie we have encountered this anger and disillusionment again and again, both in ourselves and in many other parents whose situations are similar to ours.

This is not to say that each parent of a disabled child suddenly becomes an atheist. Often the opposite occurs. The parents look to God for some reason for the situation that has so altered their lives. Some take great comfort in the belief that God knows what He's doing.

Personally I have never accepted the idea that the God described in the Bible had such tricks up his sleeve.

I have never fully embraced the concept or reality of God. But I have studied the Bible in order to understand the Judeo-Christian ethic that is the foundation of Western thought. I've studied it to comprehend the devotion and beliefs of my friends. I've studied it to try to ascertain my own beliefs and I found the Bible a remarkable book, filled with a complete moral road map and encouragement for spiritual endeavor. And I understood why people accept it completely and how they interpret God's will and God's total omniscience in every small matter concerning their daily lives.

But I disagree with that interpretation. I agree, instead, with Rabbi Harold Kushner's thesis in *When Bad Things Happen to Good People.* He says, in essence, that the God of the Bible created nature and man with all of the perfection and imperfection that naturally evolve in any living, changing organism. Just as it is inherent in man that mistakes will be made (by *man*, not necessarily by God), so it is inherent that imperfection is allowed in nature—imperfection is, in fact, an integral part of nature.

We are in awe of the four-leaf clover. Yet it is an oddity, a mistake. Some of nature's mistakes are fascinating. Some are devastating. Sometimes cells just don't separate properly and not every microscopic chromosome goes where it's supposed to go.

This, I understand, is the "nature" of nature, not someone else's God dictating how a child's life should be affected forever.

To realize this makes me less angry at the God of my friends and family.

Rabbi Kushner writes that we need to learn to forgive God for not creating a flawless world. If you believe He created man and nature, then you must also believe that He created these incredibly intricate "machines" to run on their own, mistakes and all, because that's certainly how they work. To illustrate this concept further, Rabbi Kushner says that we also need, for example, to forgive our parents when we discover that they are not the perfect human beings we thought they were. Although they never *were* perfect, we had unknowingly misinformed ourselves because we were so firm in our beliefs that we couldn't see the whole picture clearly.

Only your own *point of view* can change. Your mother, your father, and your God have always been who they are.

Painfully we grasp a higher truth—that the world works differently than we thought. But if we can thrash our way through the trauma that accompanies this realization, maybe we'll be far wiser for it.

19

Do we dare try again?

May 25. It's Memorial Day weekend and we've arrived at my
cousin Judy's in Berkeley to attend my cousin Lisa's wedding.

The drive from Los Angeles actually is supposed to take six
hours. But the swinging couple in their sports car who started that
rumor did not take into account travelers schlepping two small
cranky tots. In our case it took a neat nine hours.

Now I'm sitting in Judy's kitchen at 5:00 in the morning, unable
to sleep. I had a mad desire to get out of bed and look at my
cousin's enchanting Berkeley house. How I miss northern California! I miss it with an ache, a longing recognized only by the
natives, or semi-natives, like me. Northern California *smells* different. Like flowers. Like air. It's cold here. Clean. Green. While
lying in bed I fantasized about just staying here, not going back
home with my family.

As I wandered around my cousin's kitchen I realized with a start
that the carved antique china shelf is not a reproduction bought in
Beverly Hills but one that was truly made when it was supposed to
have been made. And the round marble cafe table I'm writing this
on is not a formica look-alike.

This house is filled with wood—wood floors, panes, furniture.
And glass. And surrounded by trees that are *not* landscaping.
They're just trees—lots of them, with no plan. There's no plan to
the house, either. Neither to the architecture nor the furnishings.
The house self-evolved and every aspect of its owners is evident in
its evolution. Crazy, eclectic spontaneity. Immediate personal
choice has won out over what "goes with" what. Somehow it is all
just right, like Baby Bear's porridge. It's nice to be here, in this
warm kitchen, quiet and alone for awhile.

June 3. My cousin's wedding was great. So was having an
adventure away from home. Now we're back. The day is beautiful, breezy, with a clear sky. So flawless a day I feel should
somehow be put to special use. But what am I doing with it?
Reading *People* magazine while, by some miracle, both my children
are napping. Eating a healthy bowl of Rice Krispies for lunch.
Thinking about chorionic villi sampling. No, this is not a term for
checking out condos in the Greek Isles. It's a new way of testing
the fetus during pregnancy to rule out chromosomal problems. It's
done by a catheter, guided by ultrasound, inserted into the uterus
through the cervix to withdraw a tiny bit of chorionic villi tissue.
This tissue surrounds the fetus and later becomes the placenta. It
can be tested, just like the amniotic fluid, but the advantage is that
it can be done much earlier in the pregnancy than amniocentesis,
between the eighth and twelfth weeks. Preliminary findings, such as
evidence of Down Syndrome, can be reported in two days after the
sample is taken. The test is new and has just begun to be offered in
a clinical setting. Before that, it was only available as part of
research projects.

CVS, as it's cozily called by its advocates, is apparently more
risky than amniocentesis in terms of possible miscarriage, to the
tune of two to four percent. A doctor at the Harbor Medical
Center in Torrance, California, does it in a clinic. Patients must
have appointments for consultations before they can be tested.

I think about those famous septuplets born at twenty-eight
weeks. I see their perfect forms photographed by *People* magazine's master invaders of privacy (and I an eager voyeur) and I
think, God, they're real, living babies. Some are ailing but they're
people. Abortion at twenty-eight weeks or twenty-four weeks or
twelve weeks is the termination of life. So why even look into
chorionic villi sampling or amniocentesis and perhaps threaten the
life of a fetus by the procedure itself? What fetus, you ask? No
fetus yet! We're still in the thinking stage but it will probably be
soon. The mere thought of another child with Down's is hard to
accept. It happens. But the thought of terminating—I can't even
say aborting—a pregnancy is also so horrible I cringe as I write
about it.

Just in the last couple of months I've found these letters in various publications I subscribe to. They tend to make one think twice about trying again.

A parent's letter from the newsletter, *Horizons of New Hope*, May/June 1985—from M. B. of Anderson, Indiana:

> One year has passed since we took our daughter, Esther, to Germany for cell therapy. We are really pleased with her development. She's almost three and attends a developmental preschool every morning.
>
> Nine months ago our second child was born, also with Down's Syndrome. I am wondering if any other families in NHPA have two with Down's and would like to correspond. We plan to begin cell therapy for our son as soon as possible. He's enrolled in an Infant Stimulation program and a class at Playful Parenting; both have helped.

✳ ✳ ✳ ✳ ✳

From "Reader's Forum," *Exceptional Parent* magazine, April 1985:

> We are parents who have never known what it is like to have a "normal" baby. Our first baby was a boy born with heart defects. We went through eight months of constant hospitalization with heart failure until his open heart surgery at eight months old.
>
> The week of his open heart surgery, I got pregnant with our second child, a daughter born with cerebral palsy, mental retardation, and a seizure disorder.
>
> My husband and I kept her at home and vowed we would never place her, but when she was six years old, the physical care got to be overwhelming. We placed her at UCP/SCF in Los Angeles. One year later she passed away from seizures.
>
> Now at the [mother's] age of thirty, we are trying to have another child. Psychologically, we are scared but after reading some of your articles we have become surer that if we were chosen again to have another child with a problem, we could handle it.
>
> We would like to hear from parents in our position. Do we dare try again?

✳ ✳ ✳ ✳ ✳

From "Spotlight on Members," *HANDS* newsletter, Marshall, Texas, June 1985:

> J.A. and D.A. have always lived in Texas. J. is from Dallas, and
> D. is from Kernes. D. is a Texas Utilities ICC Supervisor and they
> both love to travel. J. loves to cook and is involved with the
> Epilepsy Association. They have three children, D. is nine, B. is
> seven and multiply handicapped [with] profound cerebral palsy, and
> J. is fifteen months old and has Down Syndrome. They've been
> married twelve years and have been very active in HANDS since J.'s
> birth, and have helped many parents.

The letters say it all.

June 10. Max is four years old! We had a big party for him, and
he loved every minute of it. He was jumping up and down with
excitement. Sometimes I look at him and am filled with such
appreciation for his health and innate intelligence, for his adorable
face and bright eyes. But those thoughts frequently turn to longing
about his sister. I want her to be perfect too. Maybe one day I'll
stop wanting that. Maybe one day all my sadness will vanish and
how she is will be fine with me. Actually, although it's hard to
explain, in a way it already *is* fine with me. She is delightful,
bright, expressive, alert, and adorable. But I worry that as time
goes by the world won't think so.

   With my son, I won't worry about what the world will think
because he is completely able. He can fend off the world, all by
himself. As a matter of fact, the world's probably going to have to
fend *him* off!

* * * * *

I had an interesting conversation yesterday with a woman at my
son's friend's birthday party.

   Her two-year-old daughter was mistakenly diagnosed at birth as
having Down Syndrome and for four weeks she didn't know for
sure. The chromosome test came back with no indication of
Trisomy 21, but the feelings still haunt her.

   This little girl is absolutely beautiful. She has blonde hair with
Shirley Temple curls, sparkling blue eyes, flawless skin, and is as
bright as a penny.

   Her mother told me that at least once a month, when she is with
her children in a public place, such as a restaurant or mall, some

incredibly forward person will come up to her and ask her a question like "What's *wrong* with your daughter?" or "Did you have a difficult birth with her?" or "Why are her eyes like that?" Some say outright, "Your daughter is Down's, isn't she?"

I'm astounded by this woman's story. No one has ever said anything to me about Sophie and she *does* have Down Syndrome! I'm especially sensitive to seeing perfect, pretty toddler girls because I have a tendency to heave a tiny inward sigh of longing. And as I first met this child, before her mother told me this story, I thought, Some moms are so lucky—this girl is a little perfect doll!

Life is funny sometimes.

June 22. Sophie is sitting up by herself—actually getting herself into a sitting position from her crawl position. She has also started to pull herself up to her knees and occasionally to her feet.

She can climb up the step from the family room and into the kitchen and scoot around scavenging for edible tidbits on the linoleum floor. I've rescued quite a few dustballs and crumbs from her eager grasp.

Since Sophie's had the tubes in her ears, her speech development is on target. She is babbling wildly! It is such a relief to hear her "da-da's and ba-ba's." At nine months old, she is far and away above the other Down's children her age that I've met (probably a typical statement for every mother of a child with Down Syndrome).

Maybe Dr. H.'s B_6 program is partially responsible. As part of this program, Sophie will be examined and given a follow-up Evoked Potential test at one year of age. So far, all the other babies on the program have normal Evoked Potentials after a year on this program! Before this research project, babies with Down Syndrome who were tested for Brain Stem Evoked Potential showed abnormal results after about three or four weeks of age. The B_6 somehow is affecting positively the ability of the brain to receive and process sight and sound stimuli. The jury is still out on what that means in terms of development, and we won't know for at least a few years. We're hoping for any stabilizing factor in a seemingly uncontrollable problem. Actually we're secretly hoping for a miracle. Who wouldn't?

June 29. Sophie's pulling herself up to a standing position on everything! The TV, the bathtub, the couch. I don't know what I expected exactly, but with all the dire predictions I heard from doctors and physical therapists, I'm thrilled each time my daughter defies them.

Sophie's friend, Jackie, thirteen months old, with Down Syndrome, can make signs for "more," "all gone," and "duck." She can also say "up" and "ba" (for yes). She's doing so well. She's still not crawling but pulling herself up to a standing position, clapping her hands to music, and puckering up for kisses. She is a doll!

Because of their Down Syndrome features, Sophie and Jackie look a little alike. Both are petite—about the same size. Both have little pug noses and semi-oriental eyes. One day Jackie's mom, JoAnn, and I were holding our babies as we were walking out of a coffee shop. Four older ladies saw us and cooed, "Oh, how darling, what cute babies." Then one of them asked, "Are they twins?" JoAnn and I politely answered no. As we left the restaurant we looked at each other and simultaneously burst out laughing.

It's great to have a friend I can really laugh with when things like that happen.

We thought of several snappy answers we could have offered. JoAnn's suggestion: "No, but they both have the same father."

July 2. A recent letter to Ann Landers reads as follows:

> Dear Ann Landers: I just finished reading the letter from 'Down about Down's,' and I am thoroughly disgusted with the woman who wrote it. She felt that life had cheated her because her child was not 'normal.' That insensitive mother should get down on her hands and knees and thank the good Lord she has a child.
>
> My husband and I have been wanting a baby for eight years. If God sent us a Down's Syndrome child we would be thrilled. My sister and her husband have a Down's child. She is the sweetest, most adorable eleven-month-old I have ever seen. This youngster never cries. She has a golden disposition and goes to everyone in the family without a minute's fuss. I've seen her cuddled by at least fifteen different people in an evening, and she just loves it.
>
> I believe God sent us Down's children for a reason. Those special youngsters teach us so much about compassion and real love. The

gentleness of the little darlings is a model that many adults could learn from.

Please print this letter. Every parent of a Down's child will be grateful.—R.S.T., Quebec.

I didn't read the original column by the child's mother. It may have been bitter or insensitive, I don't know. But I do know one thing: that mother has a right to her feelings. Yes, she can "thank the good Lord she has a child," but there's nothing delightful about the fact that her beautiful child was born with a crooked road map over which the mother has limited control. My own daughter is the most delicious baby on earth. But then, so was my son. It is not her Down Syndrome that makes Sophie a "darling." Rather, it is the fact that she is a delightful human being! Some days, however, I want to pound my fist on the wall in anger that my daughter's life will be hindered in any way. And those feelings are sometimes hard to understand if you're not a parent in this position.

I hope that the well-meaning and loving woman who wrote that response to Ann Landers will have a house full of children one day, because she would be an excellent and caring mother. But meanwhile I say to her, "Have some forgiveness in your heart for a mother who might have a less than perfect reaction to the birth of her disabled child."

20

There's nothing to be sad about right now

July 10. Sophie is ten months old.

I've noticed something about myself lately. I've fallen in love with Sophie. I hardly ever feel sadness associated with her. One reason is that she is turning out to be such a star. She laughs all the time, is active—crawling, standing, sitting, even making a special "puh" sound for her papa. There's nothing to be sad about right now. As time goes by we will face new barriers, but for now the immediate ones seem conquered.

* * * * *

All the parents of children with Down Syndrome who told me Sophie would be wonderful were telling the truth! I thought for sure they were either trying to make me feel better or were blind to the problems of their own children. I'm so glad I was wrong. Sophie seems just great to me. More than great—sensational. I love her. I love to see her in the morning. She's so bright, alert, and responsive.

In a way I feel angry about all the horrible myths and untruths I heard and believed about Down Syndrome—that the kids were unresponsive and unable to learn, that they would be nothing but a burden. Many parents still are being told to give up infants with Down Syndrome for foster care or adoption.

The only way we could learn that those things were not true for our Sophie (or for her friend, Jackie, or for so many other kids we've met) was to live through this time and see it with our own eyes and hearts.

I have become casual and carefree with my daughter, instead of intense and worried, as I used to be. I can't attribute this change to one thing in particular, but to all aspects of Sophie's remarkable progress.

She's the best baby in the world right now.

July 12. Sophie has learned the neatest trick. We've been working on it together, and yesterday we had our first big success. When I say, "How big is Sophie?," she raises her chubby arms high above her head and I say, "So big!" And then when I laugh and hug her and clap wildly, she claps too! What a smart baby.

I don't know how this happened, and no one ever could have convinced me that it would, but I now feel that I have a baby daughter—not a baby daughter with Down Syndrome. It's as if I've opened my eyes and there she is—a real live, perfect daughter, the one I'd always dreamed about.

Yes, I am still very aware of Sophie's potential problems and work on preventing them every day, whether it's by correcting her stance, teaching her about the world, or administering her B_6 or her MSB formula. But I feel the worst part is over for now. We've done so many right things for our daughter—things that are working—that I can sit back for awhile and enjoy her. Life has returned to normal. (Or maybe I've just become used to a somewhat abnormal routine!)

July 14. Our cozy routine might be interrupted once again in about eight months. This morning I feel queasy and dizzy even though I'm only two days overdue. I couldn't be more thrilled! Pregnancy may not be the most comfortable time in my life, but I look forward with great anticipation to a happier ending this time.

I'm probably only about fifteen minutes pregnant, but already I'm pondering whether or not to have amniocentesis. I'll have plenty of time to think that over.

I just returned from a luncheon with Sophie's volunteers. Many months ago, before Sophie was moving on her own at all, I'd promised them a luncheon when she started to cross-pattern crawl. I remember saying this to them while thinking, Probably right after hell freezes over. At that time, how could I have known all the

progress she would make? This was one of the happiest promises
I've ever kept. We had a great time. The food was wonderful, and
everyone had her fill of champagne.

I held off on the bubbly because of my "delicate condition." My
home test came out positive and my due date is March 15! All the
women were as thrilled about the pregnancy as I am. When I told
them their eyes lit up as if to say, "We wish you luck! We know
this time everything will be fine." What a great group—Sophie's
personal fan club. I never knew such concerned and involved
people existed. In the past, when other parents have said, "Because
of our child's handicap we have had an opportunity to meet
incredible people," I would nod politely and think, Honey, I can
think of a million other ways I'd rather meet people.

And yet because of Sophie's circumstances, I actually *have* met
incredibly wonderful, real friends I'd otherwise never have had the
opportunity to know.

July 15. I feel so crummy this morning! I've never been pregnant
and had two young children to take care of at the same time. It's a
challenge.

Yesterday I had my first OB visit with Dr. Schoenkerman for this
pregnancy. I was glad to be in his office again, although it brought
some sad feelings to the surface. In the waiting room I looked at
an album of newborns delivered by the doctors. All the babies
looked so wrinkled and funny and fine. These days sad feelings are
relatively rare, but going back to this office was a little rough.

Dr. Schoenkerman and I discussed chorionic villi sampling versus
amniocentesis. One of the reasons I'm opposed to chorionic villi
sampling is that even though you get the results early, there's the
higher risk of miscarriage. But with amniocentesis, if you find out
there's something wrong you have to go through labor and delivery
of the fetus. The whole subject is horrifying.

✳ ✳ ✳ ✳ ✳

My mother, having grown up with Betty Grable and Vivien Leigh's
Scarlett O'Hara as her role models for beauty, always knew that,
along with intelligence and wit, a girl's passport to success included
a seventeen-inch waist and flawlessly straight legs. Although she

invariably stressed to me the "intelligence and wit" aspects of
success, at that time one little matter took immediate precedence
over brilliant academic achievement: this was the fact that I was
born with slightly bowed legs.

As a result, my mother was very concerned about my physical
development. I was promptly enrolled in ballet class. I was also
taken to a serious orthopedic hospital for monthly checkups on my
bone growth and outfitted with endless pairs of corrective saddle
shoes until I begged for my first junky pair of patent leathers at the
onset of adolescence.

At one point during this ongoing drama, I was visiting my
grandmother. I was probably wearing my newest pair of the ugliest
saddle shoes in the world, complete with changeable Thomas Heels.
I remember saying to her, "Gam, I have awful bowed legs! And
why can't I have pretty shoes like my friends?" I will never forget
her answer: "Count your blessings! Just be glad you can walk!"

At the time I thought, who cares? All I know is I'm ten years
old and my legs are bowed and I have to wear these horrible shoes
and I *can* walk so that's a dopey thing to say.

Lo, these many years later my grandmother's words come back
to haunt me.

The saying "count your blessings" has never held a special
appeal for me. I've always smiled benevolently at the speaker and
passed off the advice as sanctimonious and meaningless. Because
the fact is you can't count something you can't see. And sometimes
you can't see your blessings until you lose one. Then the search is
on.

It is small comfort to one who has lost a blessing to count the
ones remaining. I have to admit, however, that although I'm not
sure if I actually *count* my blessings now, I certainly notice them
and appreciate them more. This is not a lesson I would have
chosen to learn voluntarily, but I do have a new point of view on
the lucky, simple successes in my life: a heavenly husband, a great
family, the health of my son, my own health (the very fact that I
can *have* babies!), and the fact that my daughter's heart beats like a
bass drum, while forty percent of infants with Down Syndrome also
have heart defects requiring open heart surgery.

I am more in awe of all the things that go right. I am aware of simple miracles.

My legs are still bowed. It doesn't matter, of course, because my grandmother was right. Having movie-star legs is not a blessing I'd count over ability. Nor is it a blessing I would count over warmth, concern, interest, or personal effort. My blessings do not include perfection—at least not this year. But they do include having a fantastic family, and having life itself and all the adventures that come in that sometimes awe-inspiring and unpredictable package.

21

I feel more vulnerable lately

July 27. This weekend I've run away from home. I'm staying with
my friends JoAnn and Jay. I was supposed to go to Las Vegas with
my sister but I felt too tired from this new pregnancy. So instead
Jay and JoAnn offered an escape weekend at their house with them.

This is the first time since Max was born four years ago that I've
been somewhere without my family for more than one night. It's
great! JoAnn has a guest room with a double bed, complete with a
fluffy comforter and new lace-trimmed sheets. I feel like a queen. I
should do this at *least* once a year! Yesterday we went to the beach
all day. Jay and I walked along the pier, eating a churro and
spending too many quarters on arcade games. I won a little stuffed
bee! Jay was peeved that he didn't win anything after all those
tosses and darts and basketballs. JoAnn stayed on the beach,
watching Jackie (Sophie's "twin"). I triumphantly returned and
handed Jackie the bee. She was unimpressed, but I was proud of
my small offering.

Jackie is the cutest, brightest baby! She signs "more," "play,"
"all gone," and "Mommy, get over here." That last sign she made
up. It consists of cupping her hands together and moving her
fingers toward herself. She also says, "up," "yes," "ter," (for
water) and several other sounds which only her mother can
interpret. She is fourteen months old and doing very well. I can't
stop hugging and kissing her, especially since I don't have to change
her diapers.

It's nice being "nowhere." No one needs me! I can feel sick if I
want, or tired, or selfish, or happy, or wild. I go home today.
Although I miss my family (I had a sweet dream about Peter last
night), it's great to be away from the obligation for a while.

August 2. Right now I'm at the mall, eating some greasy Chinese
food. Sophie is getting impatient in her stroller. "It's time to go!"
she crabs in her baby language.

Pregnancy. I'm so tired, my head is about to drop right into the
middle of the steamed rice.

August 7. Sophie is napping, so I've had a chance to take a shower
and curl my hair. Peter's not going to recognize me. He's so used
to coming home to a bedraggled, tired housewife. Lately he's been
crabby because the house is always messy and usually I'm lying
down. On top of that I immediately hand the baby over to him as
soon as he walks though the door. I can't blame the poor guy.
He's been as good as is humanly possible, but even my perfect
husband has his limits.

My mom is coming from Connecticut to visit for a week. I'm so
glad! Maybe I can talk her into straightening up the house each
day before Peter comes home while I pass out on the couch.

I can't wait to take unmerciful advantage of her unconditional
devotion and demand her total slavery.

August 15. My mother was here for one glorious week. She
waited on me hand and foot, cleaned the house, took care of the
children, and even made breakfast for my husband. Peter wanted
to know if he could trade daughter for mother! Now she's gone,
however, and life is back to normal—the house is a mess, the kids
aren't dressed, I'm lying around in a semi-comatose state wishing I
were Princess Di and that any moment a handmaiden would appear
to beg me to continue to rest while she takes care of everything.

✳ ✳ ✳ ✳ ✳

Next month is Sophie's first birthday. That means it's time to go
back to Washington, D.C., to get her second Evoked Potential test
and to meet again with Dr. H. In many ways I'm looking forward
to it. We're anxious to have Sophie tested and to see Dr. H. At the
same time I dread returning to a place where I was filled with so
much sadness about my new baby.

Now that we are so proud of her and in love with her, perhaps
the return trip will be a triumph rather than a sad reminder.

* * * * *

I'm about seven weeks pregnant. It feels like seven years.

We've decided against the chorionic villi sampling. It sounds too dangerous for the fetus. As tempting as it is to have this early information, I do not want to subject the fetus to the risk. Since in all pregnancies there's already a twenty percent risk of miscarriage during the first trimester, why add to the risk?

Besides, after the birth of Sophie, I'm no longer playing the odds. And I've already had one miscarriage, so I know it can happen, right out of the blue.

August 22. I realized a few moments ago that I feel tense about this pregnancy. The fear is so subtle I haven't been able to acknowledge it, but now I recognize it. I can't seem to accept the simple joy of future birth. I just can't imagine a healthy baby. I feel I don't deserve one or am "marked." At the same time I refuse to imagine an unhealthy baby.

The fatigue that I feel at this early stage has lowered my defenses. I feel more vulnerable lately, and I'm crying more often about Sophie's future. I've written it off as pregnancy emotionalism because I can't think of another reason to be feeling this way.

Peter and I talked a lot about an amniocentesis. My latest feeling is that I don't want to have the amniocentesis at all. We started this baby and we're going to finish it, so what's the point of threatening the fetus with that somewhat dangerous process? True, the tension will be greater for us, but tension we can handle! A miscarriage or abortion we cannot.

September 1. We've had an eventful week. On Monday, Sophie was rushed to the hospital with a high fever, gasping for breath.

I had taken her into the doctor's office earlier in the day because she was having a similar breathing problem. I was terrified as I heard her crying and gurgling and trying to catch her breath in her infant seat in the back of the car on the way to his office. The doctor gave her a shot of adrenaline to clear her airways, listened afterward to her chest, and said she sounded one hundred percent better. He wanted to know how confident we felt about caring for her at home, and I said I'd certainly prefer that to a hospital stay.

He was worried about pneumonia but felt that if she could remain out of bronchospasm (the cause of her inability to breathe) and take an antibiotic and bronchodilator orally, we might be able to keep the trouble under control. I was so relieved.

Sophie was sleeping in my arms like a chubby angel and seemed much better as we left the doctor's office.

At about 9:00 P.M. Sophie woke up in respiratory distress again. Her father, who had heard about but not seen that afternoon's episode, was frantic. We called Dr. Matthew, who told us to get her to the hospital. We immediately found a trusted sitter for Max, grabbed an insurance form (we're getting to be pretty good at emergencies) and ran out the door.

A chest X-ray was the first test she got upon arrival, and then it was on to pediatrics for a blood test. We were finally able to put her into an oxygen mist tent. Every time she lay down she started to choke and cough. We tried an upright infant seat inside the tent, but she was too hysterical with fear and illness to stay in it. Finally Peter climbed right up onto the large steel crib and held her close to him, both of them together in the tent. He was kind of squished, but thank God he was there! They made quite a pair in that foggy cloud. Sophie immediately calmed down, her breathing improved, and she fell into an exhausted sleep on her papa's shoulder. She hardly awoke when the nurse gave her a shot of ampicillin for what the doctor now definitely knew was pneumonia.

It was hard to leave my baby, but Peter said he wanted to stay with her that night at the hospital, and I had to go home to relieve the baby sitter.

In spite of my panicky feelings when Sophie was having trouble breathing, I was amazed at how calm I had been throughout the ordeal. I suddenly realized why. This was a medical problem with an exact medical treatment, a good old-fashioned infection to be treated with oxygen and antibiotics. Never did I imagine that one day I would view pneumonia as nothing compared to what I was grappling with every day of my daughter's life. How I wish there were an antibiotic for that.

After a good night's sleep, I took Max to the hospital with me so I could change shifts with Peter. Sophie had slept well, and her fever was down a bit. I was relieved to see her looking improved.

She was out of her oxygen tent for a few minutes, and although she still looked pale and tired, she was almost her old self. Max thought the pediatric ward was neat and was glad to see the baby sister he loves so much doing so well.

During this whole episode Max's appetite diminished and he ate almost nothing. I mentioned my concern about this to Peter, so over lunch that day, while I was staying with Sophie, Peter asked Max why he wasn't eating.

"I'm thinking," Max answered. "I'm thinking that it's my fault that Sophie is sick."

"Why, honey?"

"Because Mommy told Grandma on the phone that Sophie caught a cold from me and then it got worse."

When Peter relayed this conversation to me later, I felt terrible for my little boy. But then Peter told me he explained very carefully to Max that it was not his fault, and that Sophie got worse colds than most babies. He reassured Max that pneumonia was different from a regular cold, that he was not in any way to blame. Apparently Max felt much better because he gobbled down the rest of his lunch without hesitation.

Peter and Max left the hospital together, and I spent a happily uneventful day and night playing with Sophie, thinking up inventive ways to keep her happy in her oxygen-tented crib. By then she could lie down comfortably but was feeling so well that she was too feisty to stay confined!

We were able to take her home the next morning. Having her home and all of us together again was great. Despite the nice nurses and good medical services, this hospitalization was an adventure I'd rather not repeat!

September 8. Sophie's first birthday party (a few days before her actual birthday) was a big success; lots of babies and older kids were there. We'd requested that each of the kids and grown-ups bring an instrument to play. What fun! It was a natural, normal day, simple and happy. Sometimes uncomplicated rituals can help to smooth life's bumpy roads. They become guideposts, lighting our way. A birth? Time for a birth announcement. A birthday? Time for a party. In our case, these predictable milestones add normalcy and simplicity in a way I never noticed before Sophie was born.

Sophie will be a year old. She is thriving, flourishing. I believe she'll be walking in a couple of months. She is physically agile and quick. She is as mentally alert and responsive as any child her age. Sometimes her physical movements, like crawling and pulling to a stand, are not as strong as her unaffected peers. And sometimes there's a beat before a response. I force myself to observe these things, but they are not as devastating as I once thought they might be.

Peter and I finally discussed the undiscussable at 4:30 in the morning the other day. We had just put Sophie back to sleep after a bottle, and we couldn't fall back to sleep. We started to talk about how to carry out her home program, which we have decided to continue on a less hectic level, and I said, "You know, no matter how hard we work on this program, Sophie will still be mentally delayed."

Peter answered, "I know. But we've got to give her every chance to reach all of her potential."

He's right. And yet sometimes I feel a frantic element in our actions. Like children playing a game, we're running from one tree to another, back and forth, hoping that any movement, any action, *anything* will accomplish progress. I know the steps of her NACD program are effective, because I've seen progress with my own eyes. And yet I still wish we didn't have to do it. Maybe one day I'll quit sighing to myself and turn back into Supermom again.

In the meantime, I look forward to our visit with Dr. H. in one week for re-testing.

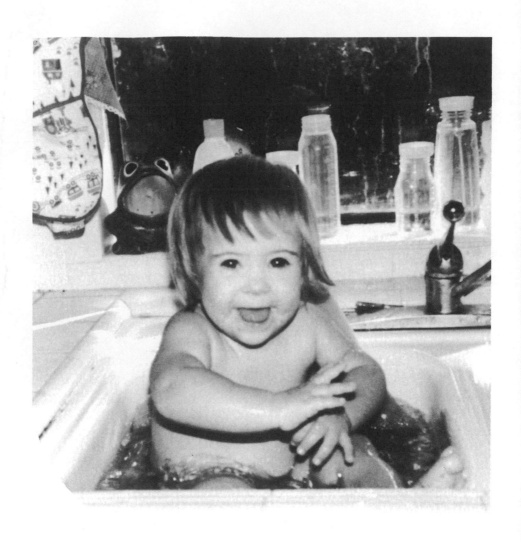

22

She will shine
as brightly as she can

September 28. We returned a couple of days ago from seeing Dr.
H. in Washington. Since we were relatively close to my parents'
house in Connecticut, we decided to make it a vacation and visit
with them for about a week too. Except for the airplane rides and
the jet lag, it was a great trip. There's nothing like traveling with a
four-year-old and a one-year-old on an airplane for five or six hours
to make you long for several uninterrupted hours on a deserted,
tranquil beach. We didn't make it to the beach; Connecticut and
Washington, D.C., were enough for one vacation.

We arranged for Max to stay in Connecticut while we flew from
there to see Dr. H. in Washington. He was excited to be spoiled by
his beloved grandma and grandpa for a day.

Our first stop was our old stomping ground, Children's Hospital.
I dreaded this part of the visit and wondered if my memories from
a year ago would bring back the same devastating feelings of grief I
experienced at that time. Just parking the car in the familiar lot
and going up the familiar ramps to the hospital entrance caused my
stomach to tighten.

Peter was holding Sophie. We were both a little tense, but
Sophie was relaxed and happy. I felt guilty knowing that we were
going to subject her to some uncomfortable moments in the hours
ahead.

As the doors to the hospital lobby whooshed open, it hit me like
a ton of bricks: grief, loss, depression, regret. I knew I was a little
reluctant and anxious, but why was I so overwhelmed at entering
that hospital? With a start I realized that I was feeling something
else—the *collective* grief of the many parents who had walked

through those doors. Mingled with the cheerful colors and antiseptic smells were the ghosts of unspoken feelings and tensions as well as endless hope in the face of the inevitable. The feelings lingered like an invisible mist. I seemed to experience much of the injustice and heartbreak that existed in the entire world at that moment, there in that one hospital for sick children. Yes, I thought, there's no point in railing against it, tearing your hair out, or beating your fists against the wall. It's simply there. It's a part of living that will always fill me with a fleeting feeling of despair. Even writing about it makes me angry. At whom? At what? I don't know. I wish I had someone to blame.

But as we took Sophie to the same blood-lab waiting room we sat in a year before, I knew we had overcome much of our initial desperation and inability to cope. We were almost cheerful with the unspoken realization that we were veterans; we could handle this.

Our confidence was somewhat shattered as the lab technician poked and poked our screaming baby's arm trying to find a usable vein. Finally she drew the necessary blood, and we hurried out of there. To see our Sophie in pain was so awful. We knew it was just a blood test, but how could we explain that to her?

We rushed up to the Evoked Potential lab for the final and most important part of Dr. H.'s research program: the Brain Stem Evoked Response test. The technician had to administer chloral hydrate, a mild sedative, to Sophie so that she would sleep during the test. I hated that but was reassured that the sedative would last only as long as a normal nap—about an hour and a half—and that there were no side effects other than some possible temporary grogginess afterward. When Sophie took the test a year ago, she was so tiny and at such a sleepy stage that she slept through the test on her own.

The technician had to place electrodes on Sophie's head. To dry the syrupy substance that makes the electrodes stick to the scalp, the technician blew cold air on each one. The whole procedure made Sophie scream, but finally she fell asleep.

After about an hour of clicking sounds and flashing lights in the soundproof room, a doctor came in to give a preliminary interpretation of the ticker-tape-style results from a computer.

First she explained that the test indicated a very minor conductive hearing loss, meaning that there was either fluid or wax or a congenital malformation in her ears, or perhaps one of the tubes had dislodged. She said this was not like the more serious hearing loss caused by affected nerves in the auditory system and was probably easy to correct. We were mildly concerned but not surprised at this, since Sophie has had chronic ear problems since birth. We were most anxious to hear about the cortical results—the brain response part of the test. How were her neurotransmitters working? Were they working normally, the goal of Dr. H.'s program?

After some detailed technical explanations of the mechanics of the test itself, the doctor finally said, "The cortical response section of the procedure has come out exactly as if it were given to a normal child."

Our hearts leaped in our chests! It worked! All those horrible mornings stuffing the B_6 down Sophie's throat, all our research, our trips and ensuing traumas were worth it! Our baby had taken a small step forward toward normalcy. To us, it was a miracle. We couldn't wait to see Dr. H. and tell her the good news!

After feeding Sophie some lunch in the hospital cafeteria, we rushed to Dr. H.'s office. She was eagerly awaiting the results of our hospital visit. When we told her that the results of the cortical brain stem test were normal, she was very happy. She is a quiet person, but we could measure her enthusiasm by the way her eyes brightened when she said, "I'm so pleased!" She examined Sophie and never stopped commenting on how alert she was, how excellent her intellectual and physical development was, and how responsive she was, even after a day of blood tests, drugs, and electrodes.

Again she asked us many questions and answered many for us. We are to continue with the B_6 for awhile. She will let us know in about a week how Sophie's blood tests came out and exactly what we should do next. As pleased as we are with Dr. H.'s work with our daughter, we are unsure if we are willing to subject her to another set of procedures again next year, should Dr. H. ask us.

But for now, we feel we have succeeded in at least one small way with Sophie, and we are deeply satisfied with that. I can't explain the magnitude of our feelings of triumph and success over the result of the visit.

September 29. While we were in Connecticut, one of my mother's teaching colleagues asked if I would speak to his class of adult students who were learning to counsel parents with handicapped children. I jumped at the chance. I have so much to say on this subject to anyone willing to listen.

My mother and I went together. I felt she could offer a unique perspective as a very concerned and involved grandmother. I often see grandparents of disabled children bringing the kids to Infant Stimulation, to speech class, or attending meetings. If my parents lived closer, they would be very active in both Sophie's and Max's activities. Grandparents sometimes do not get the credit they deserve for all the assistance and love they provide as well as total acceptance of a grandchild with problems. My parents and Peter's parents all have offered constant help, love, and support from the beginning.

My mother and I both spoke to the class, answering questions about our experiences, feelings, and adventures. Both of us talked so much that those in the class scarcely got a word in edgewise. It was so great to see these "students" (mostly special education teachers) wanting to reach out to parents. They were interested, humble, eager to learn. This experience helped to soften my attitude about special education. I'm still not thrilled at the prospect of enrolling Sophie in such a program, but at least I see there are truly good and helpful people out there. My mother and I hoped we had conveyed to these teachers that parents need to be treated with dignity and respect by the professionals into whose hands we entrust our children's health and education.

September 30. We are teaching Sophie to sign, and she made her first sign all by herself today! It was the sign for "more." Since she's such a big eater now, I knew I could use mealtime to entice her to play the signing game. For the last week or so, each time I fed her I'd say and sign, "Do you want *more*?" The sign for "more" is placing both hands together with fingertips touching. Today she made what looked like a clapping motion but then purposefully placed her fingers together. I screamed and hugged and kissed her and, of course, put lots "more" food on her tray!

She also says, vocally, "Papa" and "ball" and "bruh" (for "brother"). Max too has learned many signs, and sometimes we sign to each other just for fun. This way, when we sign to Sophie he can be included.

My initial resistance to signing has disappeared altogether, especially when I see how well Sophie's little friends can communicate, even though their speech is slow in coming. Jackie knows about twenty-five signs and is clearly delighted that she can show them all off. Signing *is* talking. I'm so glad we have availed ourselves of this option for Sophie. Of course, we also are doing many things to encourage her speech, and have for months. I'm confident she will be a big mouth.

October 1. Yesterday I was telling Max that I'm writing this book. I explained that it was about Sophie and our whole family.

"Remember how I told you we were sad when Sophie was born because she had Down Syndrome?" I asked.

He said, "Yes."

"Well," I said. "I decided to write down some things about that and about you and Papa."

"I know," he said. "I heard you talking about it on the telephone, and I know what the book is called."

"Oh!" I replied, only a little surprised that he'd heard and fully understood the conversations I'd recently had. "What is the name that you remember?"

"*Baby Sweet Bitter*," he answered, with the complete confidence only a four-year-old can muster.

I laughed and hugged him and said, "Well, that's pretty close! It's called *Bittersweet Baby*."

"Oh," he said, laughing too.

Then he asked, "Mommy, are you going to be sad when the new baby is born?"

I paused for a moment, a million thoughts going through my head. "No, sweetie, everything's going to be fine with this baby," I answered.

"Good," was his satisfied reply.

Good, I thought to myself. Now all I have to do is to cross my fingers and spit three times to ward off the evil eye, and everything really *will* be fine!

***** * * * *

We've definitely decided not to have chorionic villi sampling or an amniocentesis. We did not choose this pregnancy with conditions assigned to it. We didn't say, "We only want this baby if it has brown hair and blue eyes." We didn't say, "We only want this pregnancy if the child is perfect." We will have this baby, no matter what.

I now know I can handle more than I ever thought possible. I would not welcome the thought of another child with problems like Sophie's. That would be the second worst thing I could think of in the world—the first being a nuclear bomb dropped in my driveway. But still I know the value of that child's life would be the same, with or without disabilities.

In the game of poker you can fold when your cards are not the ones you want. But in parenting, you stay in the game no matter which cards you are dealt. The best you can do is keep throwing in nickels, practice the perfect poker face, and know that in this particular deck, the aces truly do outnumber the crummy hands. You may just have to wait a while for a royal flush.

October 9. I was reading parts of this journal that I had written almost ten months ago and I am amazed at how grief and lack of information clouded my predictions for the future. Everything is not all of a sudden peaches and cream, and we have not forgotten that our daughter was born with Down Syndrome. But I have learned so much, from books and other parents and Sophie, that I now know I was way off! My main teacher has been Sophie. She has taught me that my painful memorial service for the daughter I lost was very much a result of my own fears and sadness, not a valid prediction of what Sophie would be. I now know she is going to be so many of the things I'd thought I'd lost forever. Although concern with looks seems trivial now, she has reddish-blondish hair and will probably have an adorable freckle-filled face to go along with it. She is smart as a whip, alert, and delightful. She will join in the lunches and the gossip with the rest of "the girls" in my family and she'll probably even contribute her own gossip! She is so much more normal than not.

At just a year old, her mischievous and energetic personality overwhelms her disabilities. We know we have yet to face many serious developmental delays. We know some we will be able to control and some we will not. This will always be very hard for us to face. But with our support, the totally normal treatment she receives from her big brother (pushing, shoving, kissing, hugging, "Mom! Sophie's wrecking my toys!"), and the support of grand-parents and aunts, uncles, cousins, and friends who know her and love her (and who also know she can be a pain), she will shine as brightly as she can. And to me, *that's* what perfect is.

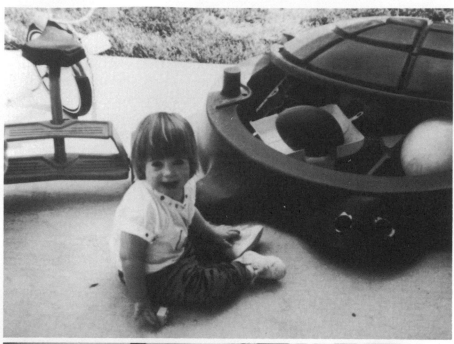

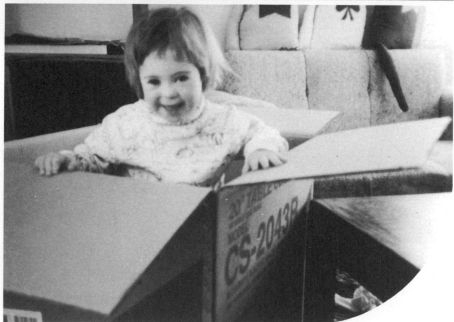

Epilogue

When Sophie was eighteen months old, I gave birth to a healthy, strapping ten-pound-four-ounce baby boy to whom we gave the illustrious name of Morrison ("Moe") Kanat-Alexander. He has brought us unmitigated joy, comfort, and many extra diaper changes. He has restored normalcy and night feeding to our home.

To those parents who are asking themselves, Shall we try again after the birth of a disabled child?, I say you must ultimately make your own decision. But for us, it was absolutely the best thing we could have done.

The philosopher L. Ron Hubbard once said something to the effect that if you feel your job is too tough, double it. This advice applies perfectly in our case. The very tough job of raising Max and Sophie was nothing compared to taking care of all three!

I am reminded of a story my Grandpa Peretz passed down to my father, who in turn passed it down to us:

The village butcher, Velfel, complains to the rabbi that his in-laws from Pinsk are coming to live with him and his wife and two children in this small one-room shack.

"Rabbi!" he wails, "How am I going to fit them all in? Surely you can ask God for more room for me and my family!"

So, the next day, after much prayer and contemplation, the rabbi returns to the butcher and exclaims, "I have just the solution!" as he proceeds to bring a cow, three goats, five chickens, and his widowed neighbor, Yetta, to live in the butcher's house, just as the in-laws from Pinsk arrive with all of their worldly goods.

"Rabbi!" cries the butcher in distress, "This is terrible! We can't live this way."

"Trust me," says the rabbi.

Three days later Velfel the butcher comes knocking on the rabbi's
door, hat in hand. "Rabbi," he begins hesitantly, "with all due
respect, my family and I are beginning to question your judgment.
My house is so crowded that we are unable to eat or sleep or even
speak to one another without interruption."

The rabbi thinks for a moment and then exclaims, "I have just
the solution!"

With a look of trepidation Velfel beseeches the rabbi, "Please,
Rabbi. We are living in the midst of your *last* solution! Surely this
one will be better?"

"Trust me," says the rabbi as they walk together back to the
butcher's crowded home. The rabbi then proceeds to empty the
house of the cow, the three goats, the five chickens, and his
widowed neighbor, Yetta.

Two days later the butcher, feeling like a man living in a
mansion, seeks out the rabbi. With a joyous expression on his face,
he says to the rabbi, "Surely God sent you to us. You have worked
a miracle. My house is larger, my family smaller, and my in-laws
more pleasant! How did you do it?"

The rabbi shrugged and answered, "Velfel, together, we can work
many miracles."

And so it is with us. With all the meals, diapers, clothing
changes, chores, classes, and tricky scheduling, it's amazing how
little space Sophie's problems seem to take up. Before the arrival of
Moe, her disabilities seemed bigger than anything else in our lives.
Suddenly they have fallen into place, into a more proper perspective. We still take her to classes (we have re-enrolled her in the
toddler class of Infant Stimulation), and we still work with her
every day on her speech, vocabulary, probem-solving, and signing.
But somehow the intensity of our preoccupation with her problems
has lessened.

I still cry. I still get that deep, sad, gut-wrenching feeling sometimes when I see a healthy baby girl about Sophie's age. I probably always will. It doesn't mean I love her any less. It simply means I am heartbroken about her disabilities. I probably always will be. But these times are the exceptions, not the rule.

By the way, Moe didn't "replace" Sophie. Fortunately, she is very much with us. She took her first step at twenty-one months, signs about fifty words and speaks several; her favorite phrase is "no way!" She is headed into the Terrible Twos with a vengeance. She is strong-willed, independent, bratty, huggable, charming, and beautiful.

You know, there is nothing good about illness or death or disability in a child—nothing good at all. But there are lessons to be learned: lessons about fairness; lessons about anger and grief and luck; lessons about change and acceptance; lessons about the untapped magnitude of your own abilities and endurance as a parent; and lessons about the *limits* of your own abilities and endurance as a parent. I didn't sign up for this class—I was drafted against my will. But here I am, probably a little better for it, a little more educated.

As for Max, Sophie, and Moe, they form a tight, impenetrable partnership, a sweet group of blue eyes and freckles and hair-pulling and screams and games and pillow fights. A completely normal family, don't you think?

About the author

Jolie Kanat graduated Phi Beta Kappa with a degree in psychology from the University of Oregon. She has been a professional singer and songwriter and appeared in the San Francisco cast of *Hair*. She and her husband, Peter Alexander, director of shows and special effects for the Universal Studios Tour in Los Angeles, and their three children, Max, Sophie, and Moe Kanat-Alexander, live in Simi Valley, California.

Resources

National Academy for Child Development (NACD)
2144 S. 1100 East, No. 150
Salt Lake City, Utah 84106
801/484-7913

National Down Syndrome Congress
1800 Dempster Street
Park Ridge, Illinois 60068-1146
800/232-6372

National Down Syndrome Society
141 Fifth Avenue
New York, New York 10010
212/460-9330

*Henry Turkel, M.D. (U-Series)
19145 W. Nine Mile Road
Southfield, Michigan 48075
313/357-5588

*Nutri Chem Pharmacy (MSB Formula)
1303 Richmond Road
Ottawa, Canada, KXB7Y4
613/820-4200

Children's Brain Research Clinic (newsletter)
2525 Belmont Road NW
Washington, D.C. 20008

Horizons of New Hope (publication)
P.O. Box 2651
Oroville, California 95965
916/589-1250

Sharing Our Caring (publication)
P.O. Box 400
Milton, Washington 98354

Please feel free to contact the author with any reactions, comments, or questions:

Jolie Kanat
CompCare Publishers
2415 Annapolis Lane
Minneapolis, Minnesota 55441

*Neither the author nor the publisher endorses or recommends any specific treatments or theories. These resources are for readers' information only.